I0440990

Clod

To

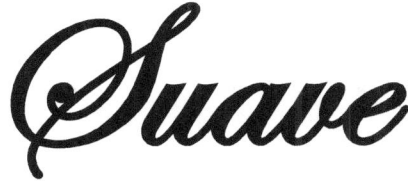

The
Etiquette, Manners, Grooming & Dressing
'Make-Over' Handbook

For

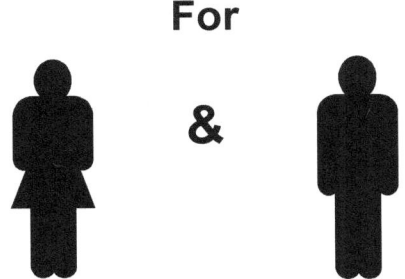

&

Michael James Stewart
Image & Etiquette Consultant

© Copyright 2010-12 by 780588 Ontario Inc.
All rights reserved worldwide.

Dedicated

To My Parents

Eileen Mary and William Gordon Stewart

who raised my two sisters,

Valerie Eileen and Nadine Mary,

and me,

in a gracious home based on manners and etiquette.

"Manners are of more importance than laws. Manners are what vex or soothe, corrupt or purify, exalt or debase, barbarize or refine us, by a constant, steady, uniform, insensible operation, like that of the air we breathe in."

– Edmund Burke

INDEX

INDEX...7

INTRODUCTION...13

DEFINITIONS 15
CLOD...15
SUAVE 15

IDENTITY 17

IMPACT 19
PERSONALLY & PROFESSIONALLY 19

ETIQUETTE 21
DEFINITION 21

MANNERS 23
DEFINITION 23

DRESSING FOR SUCCESS...25
BUSINESS – MEN [PROFESSIONAL MILIEU] 25
  Suits 25
    Fabric 25
    Colours 25
    Patterns 25
    Fitting..26
  Shirts 27
    Fitting..27
  Ties...28
  Jewellery 28
  Underwear 28
  Shoes & Socks 29
  Belts & Suspenders 30
  Topcoats, Scarf & Gloves 30
  Headwear..30
BUSINESS – MEN [PROFESSIONAL – LESS STRUCTURED].....................33
  Sport Jackets, Blazers & Slacks....................................33
  Balance of Attire 33
BUSINESS – WOMEN [PROFESSIONAL MILIEU] 35
  Suits – With Trousers or Skirt 35

Slacks 35
Blouses 36
Jewellery 36
Hosiery 37
Underwear 37
Shoes 38
Belts 38
Topcoats, Scarf & Gloves 39
Handbags 39
Headwear 39
BUSINESS – WOMEN [PROFESSIONAL – LESS STRUCTURED] 41
Sporty Jackets & Slacks 41
Balance of Attire 41
BUSINESS – MEN & WOMEN [PROFESSIONAL – LITTLE STRUCTURE] 43
Slacks / Shirt / Pullover – Applicable to men & women 43
Balance of Attire 43
Uniforms 44
Non-Uniforms 44
PLEASURE / CASUAL 47
GENERAL TIPS 48
   3.   Men 48
   Women 48
CLOTHING TIPS 49

CORRECT CARE FOR CLOTHING **51**
SUITS/JACKETS/BLAZERS/SLACKS 51
SHIRTS/SOCKS/UNDERWEAR 51
FOOTWEAR 51
OUTWEAR/TOPCOAT 51

GROOMING **53**
FACIAL HAIR 53
   Men 53
   Women 54
NOSE & EAR HAIR 54
HAIRDOS 55
TATTOOS & PIERCINGS 55
HEMLINES 55
TROUSERS & SLACKS 56

ATTIRE...56

COURTESY 57
EXAMPLES OF POLITE GESTURES 57
ASCENDING OR DESCENDING STAIRS 58
BACKPACKS 58
DOORS & ESCALATORS 59
EYE CONTACT 59
FIRST NAME USAGE 60
GIFT FOR THE HOST / HOSTESS 60
HANDSHAKE 61
HATS – INCLUDING BASEBALL CAPS, BEANIES, DO-RAGS, ETC............62
PLEASE / THANK YOU / YOU ARE WELCOME.............................62
POSTURE & BODY LANGUAGE 63
SIR & MA'AM USAGE...64
SMOKING 65
TELEPHONE USAGE – APPLICABLE TO MOBILES & LANDLINES..........66
TIMELY ARRIVALS 67
TITLES 68
    In Canada & UK 68
    In The USA...68
POLITE BEHAVIOUR 69

JOB INTERVIEWS...71
PLANNING 71
ARRIVAL AT INTERVIEW 71
ACTUAL INTERVIEW...73
FOLLOW-UP 76

WORKPLACE ETIQUETTE 77
PERSONAL WORKSPACE 77
LUNCHROOM 79
GENERAL 80

INTRODUCTIONS 83
IN YOUR HOME – UP TO SIX COUPLES 83
IN YOUR HOME – MORE THAN SIX COUPLES 84
AWAY FROM HOME – BY YOURSELF 85
AWAY FROM HOME – WITH YOUR SPOUSE.................................85
AWAY FROM HOME – WITH FRIENDS..85

AWAY FROM HOME – WITH FRIENDS – ADDING TO THE ORIGINAL GROUP 86
IN BUSINESS – INTRODUCING YOURSELF 86
IN BUSINESS – INTRODUCING ONE OR MORE PLUS YOURSELF 86

INVITATIONS 89
EXTENDING AN INVITATION 89
DATE & TIME 89
LOCATION 90
DRESS 90
ACCEPTING AN INVITATION 91

ENTERTAINING AT HOME 93

GREETING GUESTS TO YOUR HOME 97
ARRIVAL OF GUESTS – ONE TO SIX COUPLES 97
    Hosts - Couple 97
    Host – Single 97
ARRIVAL OF GUESTS – MORE THAN SIX COUPLES 98

CONVERSATION PARTICIPATION 99

SERVING DRINKS 101
LARGE PARTIES 101
SMALL PARTIES 102

TABLE SETTINGS 105
FORMAL 105
TABLE SETTINGS - FORMAL - DIAGRAM 107
TABLE SETTINGS – OTHERS 108
TABLE SETTING – BUFFET 109
CUP & SAUCER / TEASPOON 110
SERVIETTE / NAPKIN – USAGE 110
SERVIETTE / NAPKIN – RINGS USAGE 111
FLOWERS 112
NAPERY – TABLE LINEN / PLACEMATS 112
SEATING PLACEMENT 113
PLACE CARDS 113
GRACE 114
TOASTS 114
SERVIETTE & NAPKIN USAGE 115
ORDER OF GUESTS SERVED 116
ACCEPTING & DECLINING FOOD 117

Food Tip 118
When To Begin To Eat 118
Bread & Rolls – Correct Eating Method 119
Passing Items 121
Removing Something From Your Mouth 122
Asparagus – Correct Eating Method................................122
Spareribs – Correct Eating Method..................................123
Fingerbowl Usage 124
Posture..124

CUTLERY 127
General Usage 127
Cutlery Placement – When Pausing..................................129
Cutlery Placement – When Finished.................................129
Cutlery - Holding 130
   Knife 130
   Fork 130
   Spoon – Soup 131
   Spoon – Dessert 132
   Spoon – Sauce/Gravy 132
   Spoon – Sorbet 132

STEMWARE – HOW TO HOLD & USE 133

COFFEE & TEA SERVICE 134

PORT & LIQUEUR SERVICE 135

FOOD & WINE MATCHING...137
   New World 137
   Old World 137
Start with a Dish..137
Start with Wine 139
   White Wines 139
   Red Wines 139

WHICH WINE WITH WHICH SPICE? 141
White Wines..141
Red Wines 142

ENTERTAINING AWAY FROM HOME.......................143
Personal 143

ARRIVALS & DEPARTURES 145

DATING 147
THE INVITATION / WHO IS THE HOST 147
TRANSPORTATION / VENUE PROTOCOL 147
PROVIDING DATE AND LOCATION 148
FOLLOW-UP 150
HANDLING A BAD DATING RESULT 150
HANDLING PRESSURE TO BE INTIMATE 151

TIPPING 153

TRAVELLING – BEYOND YOUR COUNTRY'S BORDER 155

WEDDINGS - BRIDAL COUPLE 157
BRIDAL REGISTRIES 157
INVITATIONS 158
THANK YOU NOTES 159
ATTIRE 160
SPEECHES 160
BEHAVIOUR 160

WEDDINGS - GUESTS 163
INVITATION ACCEPTANCE 163
GIFT 163
ATTIRE 164
BEHAVIOUR 165

FUNERALS 167
OVERVIEW 167
FLOWERS OR DONATION 167
VISITATION 168
FUNERAL SERVICE 169
INTERNMENT OR INURNMENT 169
ATTENDING THE WAKE 170

INSIGHT 171

INTRODUCTION

Are you a **clod**?

Most likely, your response to that question would be, 'Absolutely not!'

Then you must be *Suave* !

Most likely, your response to that assertion would be, 'Well, maybe not quite *Suave*'.

The fact is, most people really cannot answer the question; because, they are so used to just 'doing' that they are not aware of how they are 'doing'.

The way you act and carry out functions is usually based on what you were taught, when you were young, at home and what you witnessed watching your friends.

Unless you were very fortunate, what you learned, most likely, left large gaps in your knowledge of etiquette and manners, required and expected, in the social and business world of today.

> ➤ Ignorance is not bliss! It is merely ignorance!!

> ➤ Professor Henry Higgins, of 'Pygmalion' and 'My Fair Lady' fame, asserted it was the way people spoke that kept them in their respective place in society and prevented them from rising to a higher station in life.

> ➤ It is my contention that he was absolutely correct; but, the addition of manners and etiquette, are also necessary, in order to be successful at improving how one is view by others and how successful they become.

> ➤ Even Eliza Doolittle, would never have been accepted as a Duchess had she not improved and refined her manners and etiquette.

13

➤ No matter how much money one makes, they will never truly be accepted by those around them until they obtain, and use, manners and etiquette.

➤ Whether we like to accept it or not, people judge other people by first impressions.

➤ As time passes, people continue to judge each and every thing they notice about others.

➤ Usually, people do not judge others by how they, themselves, appear or perform; but, how they think others should appear or behave.

➤ You may be the nicest, kindest, most educated and intelligent individual around; but, the more you project a lack of manners and awareness of etiquette, the less others will think of you.

➤ The perception by others, of you, has a profound effect on employment opportunities, social advancement and personal relationships.

➤ The above may offend you; you may feel that being judged, in such a manner, is unfair and discriminatory; and, on a fundamental level, you would be correct.

➤ In a perfect world, everyone would appreciate you for the inner perfection you possess and would: hire you; befriend you; or love you.

➤ Well......the world is not perfect and people exercise their perceived right to judge each other by applying basic rules of etiquette and manners.

➤ The depth of etiquette and manners one must embrace depends to what level of society you wish to aspire.

DEFINITIONS

Clod

- Awkward, clumsy, rude, unpolished, unsophisticated
- A dull, stupid person; a dolt.
- Blockhead, chump, dolt, dullard, dummkopf, dummy, numskull, dimwit, dumbbell, dumbo.
- Bimbo; Himbo.

Suave

- Effortlessly gracious and tactful in social manner.
- Smooth, urbane.
- Smoothly agreeable and courteous.

IDENTITY

Which of the definitions on page 15 do you most closely resemble?

You may identify with the definition of being awkward, unpolished or unsophisticated; but, certainly do not consider yourself a chump, dolt or dimwit. Fair enough; but how you categorise yourself only counts when you are the one who is judging. Once you step outside your door, you are being observed and judged by all around you; and, whether you like it or not, they are the ones who will make the decisions that affect everything from: being hired; being promoted; being treated with respect; finding a date or a mate; being popular or being lonely; to whether you get a seat on an overbooked plane or an upgrade on a cruise or upon checking into an hotel. In other words.....almost everything you do in life.

How you dress, walk, speak, eat, and act, affects how you will be treated by others.

Scoff if you want; protest all you want that you do not care what people think of you; demonstrate how much you do not care how others view you by acting like a boor [a person with rude, clumsy manners and little refinement; a peasant].

That might satisfy you on some masochistic level; but, deep down, unless you are a psychopath [a person with an antisocial personality disorder, manifested in aggressive, perverted, criminal, or amoral behaviour without empathy or remorse] or a sociopath [one who is affected with a personality disorder marked by antisocial behaviour], you want others in your life, and those who can have a positive impact on your life, to respect you.

IMPACT

Personally & Professionally

- For every person who feels life has treated them unfairly, there is a list of reasons why it has occurred.

- If you are lonely, having difficulty finding a job, seemingly unlucky in love, lacking friendships – you must decide whether you consciously, or unconsciously, have been the cause of your difficulties; or, have they, truly, been imposed upon you by others.

- Do you: act 'put upon'; mope around looking like you are feeling unwell; pay very little attention to your personal appearance; project an image of being a loser?

- Don't know how to act in most situations, because you were never taught.

- All of the above can easily be rectified:

  • study this manual, and put into practice what you have learned – by doing so, you will never again be able to use 'not knowing how to act' as a reason for failure in any situation;

  • correct your posture;

  • stand, walk and sit with you shoulders back, back straight and chin up;

  • change your hairstyle;

  • smile instead of scowl;

  • pay attention to what you wear – make certain your clothes <u>are clean and smell clean</u> – no one wants to associate with someone who thinks so little of themselves that they don't bother to wear clean clothing;

- shower, and wash your hair, <u>every day</u> – no matter how little money you have, you must use some of it to always have on hand a bar of soap and a bottle of shampoo;
- maintain clean hands and manicured nails – if you presently bite your nails, STOP – no one will want you touching them [in a personal relationship] or working for them when you have bitten nails;
- keep your footwear clean;
- smile – who wants to associate with someone who walks around all of the time wearing a scowl or a frown.

You may be thinking, at this point, the above might work for some people; but, it will not work in your case; because, you are: overweight, too skinny, homely, knock-kneed, bowed-legged, pigeon-toed, forced to wear thick glasses, bald, hairy, blah, blah, blah. Those are all, ultimately, excuses. The truth is, there are many successful people who face one or more of the above challenges and are successful, loved, employed, etc.

Rather than using any of the above as excuses for failure, loneliness or unemployment, they have worked with it, or around it, and come out ahead.

Jewellery, makeup, hairstyle, clothing and a smile can transform the plainest person into a bombshell!

Fuller cut trousers, or a skirt slightly below the knees, can compensate for knock-knees or bowed-legs.

Overweight can be handled by dieting [provided the spirit is willing] or with thoughtfully selected clothing, etc.

Thick glasses – hello – contact lens.

Bald for men today is no excuse. Women can wear their hair short, if it is actually thin, rather than bald; or, wear a wig.

In other words, stop blaming every possible thing, or person, and take responsibility – change the situation and you; and, your life will change.

ETIQUETTE

Definition

- a set of rules dealing with exterior form;

- a code of conventional rules of personal behaviour in polite society, which may be open to dispute;

- behaviour may be based on custom and morality;

- the practices and forms prescribed by social convention or by authority;

- being polite – possessing good manners;

- the guiding codes that enable us to practice manners;

- meant to help people get along with each other and avoid conflict;

- respect, kindness, and consideration and is the basis of good manners and good citizenship;

- the language of manners;

- the set of rules that cover behaviour in talking, acting, living, and moving [every type of interaction and every situation].

MANNERS

Definition

- an expression of inner character;

- made up of trivialities of deportment that can be easily learned if one does not happen to know them;

- personality – the outward manifestation of one's innate character and attitude toward life;

- common sense, a combination of generosity of spirit and specific know-how.

DRESSING FOR SUCCESS

Business – Men [professional milieu]

Suits

Fabric – Pure wool worsted – being a natural fibre will 'breathe' much better than, and outlast, blends. The initial investment might be slightly more; but, will result in you not having to purchase suits as frequently.

Colours – Black, Navy Blue, Charcoal Grey – should be the colours of your first three suits. Brown, Dark Green, Heather are suitable choices for additional suits

Patterns – Solid, pinstripe, Check, Glen Check (sometimes referred to as Prince of Wales check), Herringbone, Hound's Tooth, Bird's Eye, Nailhead, [Windowpane is not recommended – considered too bold]

When colour and pattern is combined, it should present a subdued, yet debonair, appearance. If it appears bold, it is advisable that you select something else.

Remember: Your suit and accessories selection will greatly impact on how you are judged, especially when it comes to determining your maturity and ability to make measured decisions. It is, therefore, better to err on the understated appearance than the overstated.

That said, do not be afraid to rise above boring and 'run-of-the-mill'. After all, if you wish to rise above your present position, you must appear decisive, unique and worthy.

Off-The-Rack

When purchasing suits off-the-rack, make certain to select from the area that is correct for your height and weight.

If you have a long upper body, select a 'tall' jacket; short upper body, select a 'short' jacket. Never allow a salesperson to sell you a suit or jacket that is meant for someone with a different body-type.

A 'regular cut' jacket is going to look ridiculous on a full-chested man or a man with long arms.

Fitting – Make certain your suit [jacket and trousers; slacks] is 'fitted' properly, by someone who is properly trained to use, 'chalk' or 'soap' and pins, to indicate what alterations the garments require for off-the-rack or a measuring tape for made to measure. If the correct series of body measurements are not done, the suit will never fit you properly.

Jacket sleeves should show one inch of shirt cuff. Trousers and slacks should be slightly angled so that the front just breaks and the back is midway down the back of the shoe heel.

Pants' cuff or no cuff is a personal decision. Consider each suit's overall appearance before deciding. Cuffs on some suits can be very smart; whereas, on others, cuffs can look quite dowdy or superfluous.

Trouser bottoms should touch your shoes at the front and be half way down the back of your of your shoe. Never allow the trousers to touch the ground.

If having a made-to-measure suit tailored specifically for you, instruct the tailor as to whether you dress on the left or the right; since that will make a difference as to the cut of the trousers' crotch.

N.B. – NEVER, and I do mean, NEVER wear your trousers or slacks so that your socks can be seen. To do so will completely undo everything you are attempting to achieve. It makes you look as if you have just survived a flood and/or you are some yokel who does not know any better.

N.B. – **In USA** – Unfortunately, there is a propensity throughout the USA for tailors and salesmen, who measure for trouser cuffing [bottoms], to do so in such a way as to cause the trousers to be too short, resulting in socks showing and the wearer appearing as though they just arrived from the farm or survived a flood.

Make certain when being measured for cuffs [bottoms], the person doing the measuring is told that you do not want the cuffs too short or for your socks to show.

Shirts

White, light blue, light grey, tan – plain, pinstripe, white-on-white, blue-on-blue

Fitting – It is often stated that you should able to fit two fingers between your neck and collar. Personally, I feel it results in a 'too loose' look. I prefer one finger allowance.

The cuff should touch the side of your hand exactly where the hand meets the wrist. It must show one inch below the jacket's sleeve. If it is too short, your arms will appear as if they are too long for your body; and, if they are too long, they will look as if you are wearing an hand-me-down.

By having both your shirt and jacket the correct length, you look professional.

Ties

Complementary to the suit; conservative yet stylish; do not undo a great outfit by wearing a 'Jack Flash' tie.

Invest in one new tie per month and, after the first year, rid your wardrobe of one per month. In that way, your ties will always appear fresh and stylish.

Jewellery

Unless you work for the mob or a brothel, less is more.

When deciding whether to wear gold or silver jewellery, take into consideration your colouring and stick to the one chosen. Do not mix the two.

No more than one ring, including a wedding ring, on each hand. If you wear a neck chain, always wear it under your shirt, even if dressed casually. Wrist bracelet, if worn, should be minimal.

In today's business milieu, an ear-stud is, usually, acceptable, as long as only one is worn and it is small. That said, before you decide to wear one to work, I think it would hold you in good stead with your employer, if you asked how the company would feel if you were to wear one at work. In most cases, the response will be positive; but, by asking, they will realise that you respect the company.

Underwear

Wear it! It simply is totally unacceptable to appear in public without wearing underwear under your clothes. The purpose of underwear is to smooth the appearance of your groin; and, at the same time, help to absorb naturally produced sweat, thus protecting the appearance of your trousers.

Shoes & Socks

Leather, black and brown, lace-up and loafers; keep it basic; fad shoe styles – higher than normal heels, long and pointed toes – are definitely not appropriate business attire.

Invest in a pair of shoe trees for each pair of dress shoe you own and use them. After removing your shoes, lightly spray the inside of each shoe with Lysol Spray. Once dried, from your sweat and the spray, place the shoe trees in the shoes and put them in the appropriate place.

Shoes should be kept polished [at least once per week] and maintained in good repair [heels and soles].

A gentleman requires only black and brown, mid-calf or longer, socks in his business wardrobe. Dark navy blue may be worn as an alternative to black socks when being worn with a dark blue or navy blue suit.

Ankle-length socks or light coloured, patterned and argyle socks should never be worn with business attire.

In casual business situations, loafers, suede, sandals, etc., are all acceptable, provided they complement the clothes.

N.B. In business, socks must always be worn with shoes. Shoes worn without socks make one look as if they are a 'lounge lizard'.

For casual wear, very casual loafers and moccasin-type shoes may be worn without socks; however, dress-loafers, even when worn as casual wear, must be worn with socks.

Sandals should never be worn with socks.

Belts & Suspenders

For business attire, one only requires one simple black and one simple brown leather belt. Select a gold or silver buckle [simple and refined] to suit your other jewellery.

Suspenders, quite simply, should never be worn, unless you work as a clown.

Topcoats, Scarf & Gloves

Unless you are working in an environment classified as 'little structure', I feel it is very wise to invest in two topcoats – a wool topcoat for winter [with a zipper lining that can be removed for late Autumn and early Spring] and an 'all-purpose' topcoat for late Spring and early Autumn.

Nothing is smarter looking than a white silk scarf worn with a black, dark grey or dark blue topcoat. It is dressy, crisp and exudes position. If you prefer something other than that, select a dark and subdued colour, either the same as the topcoat or complementary, such as a dark burgundy.

Purchase a lined pair of leather gloves [not mittens] for wear with your winter topcoat [black to go with a black or dark blue topcoat or dark brown to go with a brown or tan topcoat] and an unlined pair of leather gloves [same colours as above] to be worn with your Spring/Autumn coat.

Headwear

Many gentlemen are, once again, turning to a fedora for headwear and looking very sharp, in the process. It certainly makes a statement and, at the same time, serves a function of keeping the head warm.

Less formal, but still fashionable, is a tailored peak-cap in a solid colour to make the topcoat.

Never attempt to wear a baseball cap with a tailored topcoat. To do so would be to undo everything you are trying to accomplish. Rather than making you look 'hip', it will, simply, make you look poorly informed.

In the northern climes, a pair of fitted earmuffs, in black or brown, to match the topcoat, is quite acceptable, while being very practical.

Tip Don't forget to have each topcoat and scarf dry cleaned at the beginning of wear and once more half-way through the season.

Business – Men [professional – less structured]

Sport Jackets, Blazers & Slacks

A less structured milieu allows more flexibility. Suits, sport jackets and blazers with slacks are both acceptable.

That said, the same rules apply: select tastefully styled jackets, again within the basic colour spectrum cited above.

Take advantage of various weaves and textures to provide a quality appearance.

If wearing a noticeable weave, texture, or for that matter, a checked jacket, select a solid, complementary, colour for the slacks.

Balance of Attire

For the balance of your attire, all of the suggestions and rules, as outlined in the 'Professional Milieu' section, apply.

N.B. In some professional environments, gentlemen are being allowed to wear a suit or a jacket and slacks, without wearing a necktie with their dress shirt.

If that is applicable in your workplace, so be it; but, from time to time, I suggest you wear a tie and stand out. You will be noticed......and in a positive way.

Business – Women [professional milieu]

Suits – With Trousers or Skirt

Black, Navy Blue, Dark Grey, Brown, Tan, Dark Green – plain, pinstripe, glen-check, hound's-tooth

Carefully select jacket collars and lapels to suit your face and breast size.

For the most part, three-quarter length sleeves on a jacket look as if the jacket shrunk at the cleaners.

Full-length sleeves, usually, look more professional.

Sleeves allow approximately one-half inch of blouse to show. Never have the jacket longer than the blouse – have the sleeves shortened to reveal the correct amount.

Slacks

If your suits have trousers, feel free to wear them as slacks, without the jacket.

Follow the same colour and pattern suggestions mentioned under 'suits'.

When deciding on the correct length, <u>always</u> take into consideration what height of heels you will be wearing.

The trouser's cuff should just reach the top-side of your foot, directly above your arch. Too short and it does not look professional; too long and it looks like you do not have any feet.

<u>Never</u> wear suit trousers or slacks that wrinkle through the torso because they are too tight. They should hang on your torso in such a manner that you could take hold of them at your hips and be able to move them.

The trousers/slacks should not appear to be pulled up into your crotch.

Skin tight is not professional.

Blouses

Select both the colour and style to complement, without overpowering the suit.

Check carefully to make certain the ruffled placket down the front, or tied bow at the throat, etc., 'works' with the jacket style.

Never wear a sleeveless blouse. Doing so presents a very 'cheap' look, which is certainly not flattering.

A cap sleeve should be the bare minimum worn.

A blouse's sleeve length should always be determined vis-à-vis the length of the jacket's sleeves.

Blouses being worn with slacks alone should have more flair to them than those being worn with a suit jacket.

Consider fuller sleeves; deeper cuffs; larger bow at the throat.

Jewellery

For the most part, the advice provided in the 'Men's' section, stands up well for women.

Less is more.

When deciding whether to wear gold or silver jewellery, take into consideration your colouring and stick to the one chosen. Do not mix the two.

No more than one ring, including a wedding ring, on each hand.

Carefully consider if the outfit looks better with a showy necklace by itself, or would a finer necklace and complementary brooch worn on the suit jacket's left lapel, or on the blouse over the heart, work better.

Wrist bracelet, if worn, should be minimal.

For business, earrings should have a minimal drop – avoid big hoops, long dangling or 'glitzy' earrings, unless you work in burlesque.

Hosiery

In business, pantyhose or nylons are a must when wearing a suit, skirt or dress and should be in a shade that is more in the natural shades.

Avoid tights, especially black, unless you work in a convent.

Also, no matter how tempted you are, avoid textured or patterned hosiery, except for evening wear. It is a complete faux pas to wear textured hosiery before 6PM.

Underwear

Wear it! It simply is totally unacceptable to appear in public without wearing underwear under your clothes. The purpose of underwear is to smooth the appearance of your hips and groin; and, at the same time, help to absorb naturally produced sweat, thus protecting the appearance of your skirts, trousers and/or slacks.

A properly fitted brassiere also adds greatly to a smooth and flattering appearance.

The outline of one's brassiere and underwear should <u>never</u> be seen. [A loose sweater is much more flattering than a skin-tight one that shows the sides of the brassiere cutting into the adipose along ones sides.]

Shoes

Although it is possibly not politically correct to state, women, for the most part, improve their overall appearance by adding high-heels to whatever business attire they are wearing, with the exception of when they are required to wear casual.

Basic black and brown medium-height pumps always look perfect, no matter whether worn with a suit, skirt or trousers/slacks.

Keep it basic; fad shoe styles – higher than normal heels, etc. – are definitely not appropriate business attire.

Shoes should be kept polished [at least once per week] and maintained in good repair [heels and soles].

Hosiery – appropriate length – should always be worn.

In casual, less structured, business situations, loafers, suede, dressy sandals, etc., are all acceptable, provided they complement the clothes.

Socks should <u>never</u> be worn with heels; but, may be worn with low-heeled shoes.

Sandals should <u>never</u> be worn with socks.

Belts

A carefully selected belt or sash, in a variety of materials is always acceptable, as long as it is complementary and tasteful.

Topcoats, Scarf & Gloves

Unless you are working in an environment classified as 'little structure', I feel it is very wise to invest in two topcoats – a wool topcoat for winter [with a zipper lining that can be removed for late Autumn and early Spring] and an 'all-purpose' topcoat for late Spring and early Autumn.

Nothing is smarter looking than a white silk scarf worn with a black, dark grey or dark blue topcoat. It is dressy, crisp and exudes position. If you prefer something other than that, select a smart paisley or print silk that complements your topcoat.

Purchase a lined pair of leather gloves [not mittens] for wear with your winter topcoat [black to go with a black or dark blue topcoat or dark brown to go with a brown or tan topcoat] and an unlined pair of leather gloves [same colours as above] to be worn with your Spring/Autumn coat.

Tip Don't forget to have each topcoat and scarf dry cleaned at the beginning of wear and once more half-way through the season.

Handbags

Many business women carry just a briefcase, while others carry both an handbag and a briefcase.

If you do decide to carry an handbag, it should be modest in size and business-dressy, rather than some sporty duffle bag, which should be outfitted with wheels.

Two or three, basic-colour, quality handbags are preferable to one all-purpose sack.

Headwear

If you do decide to wear an hat, select carefully, so that you do not undo the rest of the outfit.

Business – Women [professional – less structured]

Sporty Jackets & Slacks

A less structured milieu allows more flexibility. Sporty suits and jackets with slacks are both acceptable.

That said, the same rules apply: select tastefully styled jackets, again within the basic colour spectrum cited above.

Take advantage of various weaves and textures to provide a quality appearance.

If wearing a noticeable weave, texture, or for that matter, a checked jacket, select a solid, complementary, colour for the slacks.

Balance of Attire

For the balance of your attire, all of the rules, as outlined in the 'Professional Milieu' section, apply.

Business – Men & Women [professional – little structure]

In many work environments today, the dress code is either casual, very casual or uniform [company tee-shirt and black pants or jeans, etc].

If your work place is along those lines, and you hope to ever be promoted, it does still not mean you can go to work unkempt, wearing dirty or smelly clothes or looking as if you just crawled out of bed.

Even in a relaxed environment, your appearance, manners and etiquette will have an enormous bearing on whether you are considered for a promotion. Each promotion brings you closer to top management. The decision makers will want to consider those to whom they can relate and who best represents the image that the company has spent great sums of money promoting to the public.

No matter how clever you are, you will never be considered for promotions looking dirty and/or dishevelled; nor will you be considered if you are coarse-acting, foul-mouthed or project an attitude.

Slacks / Shirt / Pullover – Applicable to men & women

A growing number of work environments are allowing employees to not have to wear a suit or jacket/slacks, yet they are still expected to present a slightly 'dressy' appearance. The combination of slacks/shirt/pullover is a smart look with a 'dressy' edge, yet still on the casual side.

Balance of Attire

For the balance of your attire, all of the rules, as outlined in the 'Professional Milieu' section, apply.

Uniforms

Even when everyone is wearing the same uniform, it is still very easy to standout as unique and worthy of being considered for promotions.

In fact, if you do not apply these ideas to your appearance, you will fade into the blur of 'the mass of employees' and management will never notice you, other than to make note of your name, so they can place it on the 'not for promotion' list.

Wear a freshly-washed shirt [tee or shirt] every day. Rotate them so you always have a fresh one for your next shift.

If it is a shirt that can be ironed, do so – if you don't know how, learn. This is part of earning your promotions and way in life.

Wash your jeans or slacks at least once per week.

If any portion of your outfit gets damaged, stop wearing it and replace it immediately.

Whatever footwear you are either allowed, or forced, to wear, keep it clean and in good repair.

Non-Uniforms

In a casual workplace, where you are <u>not</u> mandated to wear a uniform, more pressure is placed upon you to select the correct attire, than if you were told to wear a specific uniform.

Freedom from not wearing a uniform can be very challenging if you do not follow guidelines.

Outside of work, you may be a big hip-hop fan who likes to wear your jeans so low, if you were to sneeze, they would end up around your ankles; or a female who thinks your upper and lower mid-drift is the most stunning piece of flesh that has ever been tattooed and, therefore, wear skimpy short tops and shirts, shorts or jeans so low, they appear as a wide belt.

If you want to keep your job, send that message to your employers by arriving at work each day, freshly showered, your hair properly groomed and dressed in clean, proper fitting, conservative attire.

At this point, you are probably thinking, the guy who is writing this must be crazy or living in another time warp; you want to wear what you like and look the way you want to look; nobody is going to tell you that you can't.

To be honest with you, you would be correct; but [ah, yes, here comes the 'but'], only if you don't want to be hired, keep your job, or ever be promoted.

Of course, if that was the case, I doubt if you would have continued reading up to this point.

My point being, an employer who is willing to hire and pay you, expects a few things in return, such as, you will: show up for work, each and every time; not be late; arrive clean and well-groomed; do the work assigned to you, in a timely fashion; be pleasant and courteous to management, co-workers and client/customers; and, be honest.

In exchange, every pay period, you will receive payment equal to the amount promised to you when hired or promoted.

The last word of the above paragraph was included because, it is so rare that all of the job requisites are carried out by the majority of today's workforce; those who do provide their employers with the expected level of work, will be the ones who are considered for, and receive, promotions.

It is that simple!

Pleasure / Casual

One might feel that away from actual business, one can wear whatever one wishes. That assumption would be wrong; and, could bring negative results.

Pleasure/casual activities, especially if associated with business [i.e. company golf tournament, bowling benefit, etc.], is still business.

Even if you are not involved directly in a business activity, you still represent the business indirectly; therefore, you must dress accordingly.

Dress in such a manner as to not reflect poorly on your employer or yourself.

Appearing in off-the-wall attire may be fun; but, it sends a poor message, which is either, 'What kind of company would hire someone like that?' or 'I'm amazed he has a job; I sure wouldn't hire him/her.'

Can you imagine how devastated you would be, if one day you walked in to an interview for your 'dream job' and the person making the final decision has seen you before; but, can only remember the snakeskin thong you wore for the industry's fundraising beach party. You lose!

Both the type of industry you work in, and the actual business you work for, combined with how high you wish to rise within the company, must all be considered when determining the level of attention you must pay to the way you dress, and act, both during business hours and after work. No company will invest in you, and advance you, if you fail to dress and act the part.

The above may seem harsh; but, it is the way it is – accept it and act accordingly.

General Tips

1. As stated earlier, dress for the position to which you aspire and not the position you have at present.

2. Be consistent – follow the standard you set during the job interview – what they 'bought' was what they, obviously, wanted; therefore, do not let them, or yourself, down by lowering your original standard.

3. **Men** – You do not need a large wardrobe [i.e. five to seven suits (or outfits depending on the workplace) should more than suffice]. By having two to three shirts per suit, plus three to four ties per shirt, and by rotating them, you will constantly present a varied and fresh appearance.

    Women – You do not need a large wardrobe [i.e. five to seven suits (or outfits depending on the workplace) should more than suffice]. By having two to three blouses, plus a few silk scarves, for each suit, and by rotating them, you will constantly present a varied and fresh appearance.

4. Remember to follow the purchase/replace/discard schedule put forth earlier. Obviously, if you invest in worsted versus blend material for your suits, they will stay in good appearance for a longer period; therefore, you can at least double the replacement periods outlined. No matter what you purchase, as with all items, refreshing your wardrobe on a rotational basis will guarantee you always look first-rate.

5. One to two pairs of both black and brown shoes is all that is required.

6. Just remember, it is not about the amount of money you spend; but, how you end up presenting yourself. Attractive, stylish and professional clothing need not cost a fortune. Shop carefully; take your time – don't go about the process in a rush; if you find a store that offers good value on apparel that fits your needs, find a knowledgeable salesperson and use them each and every time you shop in that store; ask for their advice and tell them exactly for what you are shopping and the amount you have budgeted for this visit; stick to that amount; ask for discounts – if you don't ask, you won't get.

7. If you reside in a country that allows you to deduct charitable donations, always donate your discarded cloths to a charity that is willing to provide you with a receipt. You might as well benefit from your act of generosity.

Clothing Tips

1. Always dress within your budget; but, always one level above your position expects [in other words, do not try to compete with the company President, unless you are the Vice President].

2. Keep your wardrobe fresh and current by adding a new suit every four months. Add a new shirt and tie at least every two months. Each time you add a suit, retire the one suit that is the 'most dated' or 'most worn'. The same applies to shirts and ties. Shoes should be polished at least once per week; repaired as needed [do not let the heels wear too far down]; and replaced at least once per year.

3. Dry clean your suits regularly; and, in between lightly spray the inside of the jacket, especially the armpits, with Febreze.

4. **Important Tip** – At the very beginning, purchase an inexpensive recipe file box and a supply of appropriate cards. With each and every purchase – yes, even each batch of socks and underwear – fill out a card with a basic description [upper left corner], date purchased [in upper right corner], where you purchased it and the price.

   Group the cards under headings – i.e. shirts, suits, slacks, tie, socks, underwear, shoes and topcoat.

   If the item can be dry cleaned, mark on the card the date each time you have it dry-cleaned.

   Once per month, review the cards to make certain when the dry-cleanable items were done and act accordingly. The card file will, also, help you to know when it is appropriate to discard the items.

CORRECT CARE FOR CLOTHING

Suits/Jackets/Blazers/Slacks

Before hanging up all of the above, give a quick spritz with Febreze following each wearing. Make sure to spritz each jacket armhole [inside the jacket].

Allow all of the above to dry from body sweat and Febreze before hanging them in your closet or wardrobe.

Shirts/Socks/Underwear

No matter what you have been taught, shirts, socks and underwear are all one wear items. Once removed, they go into the hamper [dirty clothes bag or hamper] for laundering.

Footwear

Always give a light spritz of Lysol Spray into each piece of footwear after being removed. Let them dry, from both your sweat and the Lysol Spray, before putting them away.

Purchase and use a pair of shoe trees for each pair of dress shoes [men and women]. They will keep your shoes looking better, longer.

Regularly worn shoes should be polished once per week.

If leather footwear develops salt marks, use white vinegar on a paper towel to wipe the salt marks away.

Outwear/Topcoat

Dry clean at the beginning of the season you will be wearing it and again half-way through the season. In between, every so often, give it a Febreze spritz, both inside and outside the coat.

GROOMING

Definition: To care for ones appearance; to make neat and trim; to do so carefully in front of the mirror.

Actually, the definition speaks volumes. Unfortunately, many people today appear in public looking like an un-made bed and then wonder why they are not being hired, promoted or asked out on a date.

Ones' appearance is all that many may judge, especially before they get an opportunity to see the person's other qualities, before getting to know the individual. Using that criterion, many never get beyond that first judgement.

As stated in the definition, appearing neat and trim are the basics of good grooming.

Unfortunately, although it says that you should groom in front of a mirror, many people don't actually see themselves in the mirror the same as others see them.

It is, therefore, important to look very carefully at those who work in your area of employment, to assess whether others, working in that field, actually do what you want to do, prior to you proceeding. Otherwise, you will make a mistake that, quite possibly, is irreversible.

Facial Hair

Men –if facial hair is worn, keep it clean and trimmed neatly. Tweeze curly or extra-long eyebrows and thin and shape them if your eyebrows look like a hedgerow.

Long sideburns are not attractive unless you are a contract killer; and, a Captain Ahab styled beard was not attractive on him; so, why would it look good on you?

Women – shape and tweeze your eyebrows to make them suit your face and leave it at that. Shaving or waxing them completely from your face never looks attractive; instead, it gives the appearance that you are tough and unsavoury. Perfect if you are a wrestler; otherwise, forget it.

Under no circumstances should you EVER have your eyebrows or eyeliner tattooed. Even the WWF would give second consideration to hiring anyone having done that.

Nose & Ear Hair

Although usually more of a problem for men, women do have to be vigilant as well about noticeable nose and ear hair. On a regular basis, follow the information below and maintain a good appearance. Allowing nose and ear hair to be visible is inexcusable and reflects very poorly on anyone who has it showing.

NEVER tweeze nose hair. Due to the presence of germs and bacteria in your nasal cavity, tweezing or pulling hair from your nasal cavity could lead to a staphylococcus infection, which could reach your brain within minutes; and, could lead to death. Nose hair should only be cut with proper scissors made especially for nose hair or an electric nose hair trimmer, which is safe and provides a good result.

Ear hair may be tweezed, trimmed or shaved.

Hairdos

Extreme hairdos, on men or women, will always stand out, but, in a negative way. Wearing a Mohawk will, most likely, mean you will not be put on the promotion list for CEO; because, as attractive as you may feel you looked, it will call into questions, by others, as to your suitability to make good judgement decisions for the company.

Tattoos & Piercings

Think before you act! That even applies to decisions you may want to make when still quite young. The giant ear-lobe plugs, the bone through your nostrils, the split tongue, the ten rings along your ear cartilage, the Maori tattoos swirling on the sides of your head, that meet in the middle of your upper lip, – those, regrettably, will consign you to a rather menial job, no matter your education level. The reason being, someone with the same education, lacking your visible artistry, will be given the job.

Hemlines

Women, when wearing skirts or dresses, should avoid trendy ups and downs with hemlines and maintain the proper business skirt lengths. Mid-knee to one or two inches below the knee is not only the most flattering length for women; but, the most appropriate for business attire.

It is a very rare woman who has legs that actually suit a mini-skirt. Sorry; but, that's the truth. Unfortunately, rightly or wrongly, wearing a mini-skirt does not add to a woman's professional credibility. It may attract a co-worker who is looking for a bit of 'slap and tickle'; but, it will not impress those who decide promotions.

Trousers & Slacks

For Women & Men – properly cut suit trousers and slacks are an imperative. They should be tailored so they are not drawn up into your groin. Wearing tight-fitting trousers and slacks for business is very unprofessional.

Attire

Much has been said about what to wear while at both work and play. The best guide to use is to ask yourself: 'How would I feel if my employer, priest/rabbi/minister/imam, parents or a potential spouse were to see me dressed the way I am?' Also, 'Does my attire reflect who I really am and what I aspire to be?' 'Will others respect me, after they see how I am dressed?'

If the answer is 'yes' to each question, then most likely, you are properly dressed for the situation at hand.

Ultimately, good grooming is all about exercising good judgement, when deciding all aspects of your appearance.

N.B. Lately, for some unknown reason, some women have begun wearing sequins and bejewelled tops, lacy skirts, lamé tops/skirts, net skirts and other eveningwear, during the daylight hours, and even to work.

Unless one is the company strumpet, such choices, before 6PM, are completely de trop and reflects very poorly on the perpetrator.

COURTESY

Courtesy is the application of manners and etiquette towards another person, or other persons; and, consists of a polite gesture, or a series of polite gestures, which then becomes polite behaviour.

By following the contents of this 'Manual', you will be courteous and known to demonstrate polite behaviour.

Examples of Polite Gestures

- Standing when someone older, or above you in responsibility, enters the room, especially, though not only, if they are female.
- Offering your seat to an older person or someone who is disabled.
- Offering to help someone without being asked.
- Refrain from saying negative things, especially about others.
- Do not be afraid of paying others a compliment; but, only if it is warranted and sincere. False compliments are nothing but flummery; and, people will realise it and resent you mocking them.
- Refrain from using swear words during general conversation.
- Modulate the level of speaking to suit the situation. In general, do not yell or feel you need to speak loudly in order to stand out.
- Respect others and their space.
- Allow others to have opinions and respect their right to differ. Just because they may differ with your opinion does not mean they are stupid anymore than you are smarter.

- Control your temper. You do not have a right to have 'temper tantrums' and expect others to tolerate them. When you act as a civilised adult, you will be treated as one.
- Ultimately, treat everyone in the manner you would like others to treat you. Your actions will come back to you many times over.

Ascending or Descending Stairs

In most countries, it is quite proper if a gentleman allows the lady to ascend the stairs ahead of him; and, to precede the lady if descending the stairs.

The only exception to this, that I am aware, is in Denmark, where it is the complete reverse. A gentleman precedes ascending and follows descending.

Backpacks

The proliferation of backpacks has been accompanied by a complete loss of respect for other people and the space they occupy.

In a crowd, such as queuing for public transit, on public transit, entering an elevator, using a revolving door [I have actually witnessed people getting their backpack caught in a revolving door and then looking surprised – duh], etc., the correct action is to remove your backpack and carry it in front of you. In that way, you will know exactly where it is vis-à-vis yourself.

On your back, you have not a clue where it is; therefore, you are, most likely, banging into people around you every time you move. You only pay for one space on public transit and do not have the right to bash into others because you are too lazy or thoughtless to carry your backpack.

Doors & Escalators

Hold the door open for the person behind you. When it is done for you, you so appreciated it; so, why not think of the person behind you and how much it will mean to them. Make their Day!

Standing to the right [or left in the UK and other countries where they drive on the left] on an escalator, if you are not climbing, is both a courtesy and fairly basic thinking.

Certainly you have the right to stand still and not climb; but, you do not have the right to impede everyone else. Allow everyone else to decide for themselves as to whether they will join the group on the right who are allowing the escalator to lift them the entire distance or join the group on the left side who are climbing along with being lifted.

If you are towing something behind you, or pushing something in front of you, either stand to the right or take the elevator, if available.

Eye Contact

Cultures vary greatly when it comes to making eye contact. Having lived in the Caribbean for many years, I learned very quickly that people in that region of the world are definitely not meaning to be rude when they fail to look you in the eyes, when speaking with you.

Their culture feels that it is rude to do so and, on some islands, you are trying to steal their soul if you do stare into their eyes.

Throughout many other cultures, certainly throughout North America and Europe, it is considered rude, and a sign that you are not trustworthy, if you do not look the other person in the eyes, when you are speaking with them.

It is very difficult for an Islander, who moves to North America or Europe, to change that habit and look into the other person's eyes. Because most North Americans and Europeans are not aware of this trait, many interviews end up not going well because the interviewer senses the interviewee is not honest or is not paying attention.

When a North American or European moves to the Islands, they must learn to change, because they are now the newcomers and must learn to respect the local culture.

First Name Usage

In spite of the supposed casualness of the times, it is presumptuous, rude and disrespectful to call someone older than you, or someone in authority, by their first name, unless they give you permission.

It is neither demeaning nor debasing to pay respect to others. One may never deserve to receive respect until they are prepared to give it; and, that respect starts with your elders and people in authority.

Mr., Mrs., Pastor, Reverend, Rabbi, Father preceding the person's last name is always correct.

If a person suggests that you call them by their first name, then thank them and, hence forth, proceed to do so.

Gift For the Host / Hostess

In Canada and the USA, bringing a bottle of wine [chilled if white] is always correct and appreciated. If wine is presented, the host is expected to serve it, either prior to the meal or during the meal. Should they fail to serve it, the presenting guest will feel, rightly or wrongly, that their choice in wine was not correct.

The same holds true if the arriving guest presents a box of chocolates. The host should offer them to everyone <u>after returning to the living room following dinner</u>. Not to do so, would indicate the host was not pleased with the selection or that the host considered them to be inferior and not worthy of being offered.

<u>The only exception</u> to this, that I am aware, is in Denmark, where it is the complete reverse. If the wine or the chocolates were served, the presenting guest would feel that the host did not like what was brought and wanted to get rid of it by having others eat or drink it.

An alternative to wine or chocolate, although becoming less popular, would be cut flowers or a potted plant.

Handshake

In social situations, especially, but, life in general, it was always the practice not to attempt to shake a woman's hand unless she offered her hand first. Today, for the most part, that has completely changed.

Certainly, in business, if the occasion calls for handshakes, then do so, whether it is with a woman or a man.

In a social situation, assess each situation and proceed with what your sense is of the moment.

If the situation calls for an handshake, and you are outdoors and wearing gloves, a gentleman should always remove their glove, on their right hand, before offering it for shaking. A woman does not have to remove her glove; but, if it involves business, then I feel it is quite proper for the woman to, also, remove her right glove, prior to shaking hands.

N.B. As mentioned in another part of this 'Manual', most Orthodox Jewish women and most Muslim women do not shake hands with men.

Hats – including baseball caps, beanies, do-rags, etc.

Unless you belong to a religious sect that insists on men wearing something on their heads while indoors, NEVER, and I absolutely mean, NEVER wear your hat indoors.

To wear a hat indoors, even within your own home, is cloddish, boorish, gauche, rude and offensive to everyone else.

When I say indoors, I mean anywhere indoors, including restaurants, aircraft, trains, schools, and any other indoor place of which you can imagine.

Please / Thank You / You Are Welcome

Always use 'please', 'thank you' and 'you are welcome at the appropriate opportunities.

'May I' should always be followed with the words, 'Thank You'.

A request for something should never start with, 'Give me'. 'May I, please, have......' is the proper way to make a request.

When someone does <u>anything</u> for you, it is proper to say, 'Thank You'.

When someone says 'Thank You' to you, the only correct responses are, 'You are welcome' or 'It is my pleasure'.

From the service industry today, all too often, when a customer offers a, 'Thank You', to the clerk, waitstaff, taxi driver, bus driver, or similar people, they receive, as a response, 'Aha', 'No problem' or 'Okay'.

Never, is such a response acceptable. It is so rude as to be offensive. In essence, such a response means: ['Aha'] 'Whatever'; ['No problem'] 'It might have been a problem for me to do that for you but I don't mind this time'; or, ['Okay'] 'Oh, did you say something?'.

When someone is polite and thanks you, respond by being polite and say, 'You are welcome'.

Posture & Body Language

One might wonder why this subject is included in the 'Courtesy' section, or, for that matter included at all.

How one holds oneself sends a strong message to those around as to how they are considered.

Slouching while listening to someone sends the message that you really don't think much of them and could not really care what they are saying. In turn, your slouching will affect how those around you treat you and react to what you have to say.

If you slouch in school or at work, you may be seriously affecting your grades or possibility for advancement; because, slouching indicates you just do not care; therefore, if you don't care why should your teacher of employer?

The same holds true throughout your daily routine, whether at home or amongst others.

Standing with your shoulders dropped and head down clearly projects you suffer from low self-esteem.

Crossing your arms across your chest, sends a clear message of: keep your distance; I don't believe you; I don't like you or leave me alone.

Placing both hands into your trouser pockets indicates you are somewhat lackadaisical, and quite possibly bored, about what the other person has to say.

Placing your hands on your hips [one or both] sends the message that you feel superior to the other person and you are daring them to challenge you.

When standing, keep your shoulders back, chin up and parallel to the floor. Hold your hands at your sides or softly clasp them in front.

When sitting, sit up straight, with your feet either crossed at the ankles or parallel to each other and your legs at right-angles. Hands should be folded in your lap.

Sir & Ma'am Usage

Several years ago, just after I began working at a new place, I was ordered to stop using Sir and Ma'am when addressing my superiors and customers. Management asserted that it was demeaning and sexist to women, using Ma'am to address them.

Obviously, I immediately refuted their claim and proceeded to explain that it is used by people outside of the 'southern USA' as a term of courtesy and respect. In fact, from infancy I was raised to use 'sir' and ma'am' as a way of showing genuine respect; therefore, throughout my life, I have done exactly that.

As a point of interest, when I attended a state dinner in honour of Her Majesty Queen Elizabeth The Queen Mother, everyone used 'Your Majesty' the first time each guest addressed her, then reverted to 'Ma'am'. So, if it was correct, and not demeaning, to use while addressing a Queen, I am quite positive it is most appropriate when being used with all other women.

If, as a woman, you are presently not comfortable being addressed as 'ma'am', I respectfully suggest you revisit the subject.

Smoking

Do not smoke around those who are non-smokers.

Most smokers, today, have become much more considerate of those around them who are non-smokers. That said, it is important for smokers to maintain an awareness of what is happening with their smoke.

Many municipal smoking By-Laws establish a specific distance from all entrances that smokers must respect. [In the City of Toronto, smoking is prohibited within a nine (9) metre radius of any entrance or exit.] In spite of those by-laws throughout the world, smokers continue to cluster around entrances, including hospitals entrances.

As stated at the beginning of this section, Courtesy is the application of manners and etiquette towards another person, or other persons; but, in the issue of smoking in the wrong places, it surpasses **Clod** To *Suave* and becomes a health issue. No one has the right to impose upon others something that will jeopardise the other person's health. Smoke if you wish; but, do it where it does not endangers others. That is the *Suave* thing to do.

Telephone Usage – Applicable to Mobiles & Landlines

Answer the phone promptly; don't keep others waiting while you light a cigarette or saunter to answer it.

If selecting a special ringtone for your mobile, remember its' only purpose is to notify <u>you</u> that your phone requires answering. Overly loud, dramatic, ringtones serve only one, logical, function; and, that is to tell others you are in need of everyone looking at you because you are pathetic, lonely, insecure, self-centred, with no regard for anyone else.

Using your mobile while someone is serving you, whether in a store, at the hairdressers, etc., is the ultimate in rudeness. There is absolutely no excuse for such behaviour. Once again, the only message you are sending, besides saying, 'I think the person serving me is of no value', would be to say to everyone around that you are, once again, in need of everyone looking at you because you are pathetic, lonely and insecure.

Also, as totally inexcusable behaviour, is to carry on a conversation in such a loud voice as to let everyone around you privy to the contents. It is your call; not theirs. No one cares about what you are saying to the person at the other end of your call. If the other person cannot hear you, adjust the phones volume, not your voice.

If you are indoors attending an event, whether a concert, movie, dinner, touring a museum, etc, either turn the mobile off or put it on vibrate. If it rings and you are expecting an important call, excuse yourself and go to a lobby area <u>before</u> answering it or calling back. Otherwise, <u>do not answer it</u>. Those around you have paid their money to be where they are and you have absolutely no right to interfere with their enjoyment; therefore, either disregard the call or go to the lobby or outside before answering. Remember, the message sent to others in the previous paragraph is the same one they will receive from the above situation.

Texting has become endemic. Texting while you are with others, or walking along the street, even if by yourself, sends a very clear message that your life is so pathetic that all you have left is to be communicating with someone else who is equally pathetic; or, you feel those with you, or around you, are boring. That may not be fair; but, it is what others think. Save your texting for times when you are alone, not walking along the street, driving or with others.

Timely Arrivals

There are no excuses for disregarding the time provided you by the Host of a get-together, whether it is casual, dressy or formal.

7:00PM on the Invitation means exactly that. A fifteen minute leeway is quite acceptable – that is, 6:55PM [absolutely no earlier] to 7:10PM [absolutely no later].

In other words [I'm spelling this out because of too many people misinterpreting what is allowable], no matter what time you are provided for the arrival time, no more than five minutes before or ten minutes after that time is acceptable.

Some Hosts will state, 'Cocktails at 7:00PM – Dinner at 8:00PM. That does not mean you can show up any time between 7:00PM and 8:00PM, even if you are not interested in having a cocktail. Either accept the time the Invitation is being called for or decline the Invitation.

When an Invitation for a party states 7:00PM – 9:00PM, it means that it is a Cocktail Party and you may 'drop in' between those hours.

That said, it does not mean you can arrive at 8:55PM and stay for two hours. If you want to have a prolonged visit, then arrive early enough to accommodate your wishes.

Unless the Host specifically asks you to stay past the pre-announced time for the event to end, you should definitely depart prior to the designated time.

Titles

When speaking with anyone with a title, use the title; after all, they have earned it. If you are not certain what the correct title is, or how to use it, ask.

In Canada & UK

The Queen = Your Majesty [the first time] then Ma'am
Governor General = Your Excellency
Prime Minister = Prime Minister [last name] or just Prime Minister
Premier = Premier [last name] or just Premier
A Cabinet Minister = Minister [last name] or just Minister
MP or MPP = Mr., Mrs., or Ms
Senator = Senator [last name]
City Mayor = Your Worship [never Mr. Mayor]

In The USA

President = Mr. President or President [last name]
Department Head = Secretary [last name] or Mr. Secretary
Senator = Senator [last name]
Congressman = Congress[man][woman] [last name]

Polite Behaviour

Following what is stated in this 'Manual', and generally acting in a courteous manner, results in 'polite behaviour'.

It will positively impact on how others see you and treat you; and, I guarantee, will, positively, affect your chances for advancements in employment.

JOB INTERVIEWS

Planning

When preparing what you plan to wear, you should take into consideration that the hiring process for most jobs will involve two, three or even four meetings. Spend time planning your complete outfits for the full interview process; and, follow the recommendations taught in this 'Handbook'. Dress to get the job.

Remember, the very first impression of you, as seen by the interviewer, will occur within the first five to ten seconds, and will carry the most weight. Dirty or bitten nails, unpolished shoes, soiled or un-pressed suit, socks that show legs, a necktie improperly tied, hair poorly maintained, poorly groomed facial hair, an un-ironed shirt [even a permanent press shirt looks better being ironed], or too much jewellery, can negatively impact on the first impression you make.

Never wear cologne or after shave. Rather than add to your appearance, it detracts from you. Allergies abound; imagine if your interviewer is allergic to scents; or, the company has a 'No scents' workplace environment rule.

Arrival At Interview

Arrive ten minutes early and go directly to the washroom. If you are wearing a topcoat, remove it.

Check yourself in the mirror very carefully to make certain you do not have mud up the back of your legs [if it is raining or slushy outside] or lint or pet hair on your suit [jacket and trousers].

If you have worn boots/ protective footwear, remove them and place them in a grocery bag, or a proper boot/shoe bag, you have brought with you from home.

Check your shoes and buff them with a paper towel, if they need it.

Check you hair.

If wearing makeup, check it and touch it up, so that it looks fresh.

Check your smile to make certain you have nothing stuck between any teeth.

Use a breath strip if you have any doubt about your breath.

You have no way of knowing how long the interview will last; and, being somewhat tense, you may find yourself needing to use the washroom during the meeting; therefore, go to the toilet.

Wash your hands.

Place your coat over your <u>left</u> arm [so that your right hand is free for shaking hands]; use your left hand to carry the footwear bag, if you used one; and, also carry your briefcase, if you have one, with your left hand.

All of the above should take no more than five minutes.

<u>Enter the appropriate office five minutes before your appointment</u> [no earlier]; proceed to the reception desk or whoever appears to be the first contact; when they acknowledge your presence, smile and state, in a pleasant voice, "Good morning [or afternoon], I am 'your name' and I have an appointment with 'the person's name'."

Listen carefully to what the person says and respond accordingly.

If they do not instruct you where you should place your coat [a boot bag], ask, "Where would you like me to hang my coat?" Then hang it, where instructed [if you have a boot bag, after you put your coat on the hanger, loop the strap over the crook of the hanger and then place the hanger where it belongs].

Listen carefully for further instructions to either be seated or to proceed somewhere.

Actual Interview

When the Interviewer is ready, you will either be told to proceed to the appropriate office; shown to the office by the Receptionist or the Interviewer's Secretary; or, the Interviewer will come to the reception area to meet you and lead you back to their office.

No matter which alternative occurs, make certain you remember to smile and thank the Receptionist.

If the Interviewer's Secretary comes out to lead you to the Interviewer's office, unless the Secretary offers their hand to shake, do not attempt to shake their hand.

The first opportunity to shake the hand of the Interviewer, whether out in reception or in their office, smile, extend your hand and say, 'your first and last name, it is very nice to meet you."

Wait for them to instruct you where they want you to sit and then wait until they have either made their way back around their desk to their chair, or are ready to sit on some other chair. Sit as they sit.

Fold you hands in your lap [<u>do not fidget</u> with your hands]; or, rest your arms on the chair's armrests.

During the meeting do not cross your leg by placing the ankle of one leg onto the other leg; merely keep your feet on the floor or cross them at the ankles.

If the meeting is prolonged, once in a while, to relieve stress, you may cross your legs but only one leg crossed over the other at the knee, allowing the crossed leg to hang parallel to the other.

Pay close attention to every word the Interview says; ask for them to clarify any question about which you are not clear.

Maintain a happy countenance, without sitting there with a silly grin on your face. You want them to sense that you are a pleasant person, not a blithering idiot.

If the Interviewer asks if you have any questions, make certain you ask any questions you have. This may be your last opportunity.

Presuming the job's salary range was included in the advertisement, do not waffle if asked what salary you are looking for. Simply state that you took note of the salary cited in the advertisement and responded to the ad because it was within your expectations.

If the salary was not mentioned in the advertisement, respond by saying at this point you feel it is somewhat premature to be discussing salary, since there is quite a bit more to discuss on both sides before that point becomes relevant.

If they become insistent, state clearly what your expectations are and do not make it sound as if you are begging. Better you lose the job because you feel you are worth more than they are willing to pay, than to let them waste the time of you and them, by having you back one or more meetings, only to discover you want more than they will pay.

Also, don't underestimate your value. If they see in you the qualities you know you possess, they will be willing to meet your expectations.

Not receiving what you feel your true value is, will lead to you being unhappy; and, therefore, not a very good employee. You and the company will lose.

Unless they raise the subjects of: Vacation; Benefits; Sick Days; Time-in-Lieu; Overtime; Expense Account; Car Expense; and, Health Insurance, do not raise them, especially at the first meeting. Presume they have those items covered and leave them for the meeting when they offer you the job.

Also, when they ask you to tell them about yourself, they are asking you about you, vis-à-vis your work, and not about anything personal. **NEVER** discuss your family, marital status, age, number of children, religion, personal health issues, where you live, your favourite singer or anything at all of a personal nature.

Never discuss conflicts with past employers or fellow workers; and, do not enquire about other jobs that may be open in the company or about the company's promotion policy.

You are there to discuss only one thing: the specific job and your qualifications as they pertain to filling that position.

When the meeting is finished, stand, shake the Interviewer's hand; and, sincerely, thank them for giving you this opportunity [even if you were not offered the job or you declined the job]. If you are to return for another meeting, still thank them for this meeting and tell them you are looking forward to the next one.

Remember to close their office door behind you.

Proceed to the Reception area; retrieve your coat; smile and thank the Receptionist, once again; and, then depart, closing the door behind you.

Follow-Up

Unless you were offered the job at that meeting, as soon as you get home you should either write a note, or send an email, to the Interviewer thanking them for the opportunity you were given. Whether you were told that you were not suitable, or that you would be hearing from them, still send the note. You never know what is down the road. Even though you may not get the job today, years later, another opportunity may arise and your earlier gesture just might make the difference.

WORKPLACE ETIQUETTE

Personal Workspace

The appearance of your workspace is a direct reflection of you. Those, to whom you answer, those whom answer to you, and your peers, will all judge you on your personal appearance, as well as your personal workspace.

Clutter does not indicate that you are a hard worker. It indicates you are disorganised. Stacks of files, whether active or not, sitting on your desk, or piled around your workspace, sends a message to everyone that you cannot keep up with your workload.

1. Maintain a clean, uncluttered and orderly work place, whether it is just a desk, cubicle or separate office.

    Whether or not cleaning staff maintains your space, invest in a roll of paper towels and a spray bottle of Windex. That is all you need to keep your space looking fresh.

    At least once per week, spray and wipe your desktop, computer [front, back and underneath, plus cords].

    If accessible, check the front of your desk for marks and remove any [if there are chairs close to the desk front, sometimes people using them will cross their legs and accidently scuff the front with the shoes].

2. Keep your desktop 'stack' free. If you are not, presently, working on a file, put it in a desk drawer.

3. Minimise desktop clutter by keeping extra pens, pencils, etc. in a desk drawer.

4. Under no circumstances, whether allowed or not, put up posters [unrelated to your work], cartoons, photos, etc.

5. NEVER, EVER, chew gum while at work, even if it is allowed. At best, it appears that you are still finishing your meal; at worst, that you are chewing your cud!!!

   Whether you chew gum with your mouth closed [obviously the only way to do it]; or, with your mouth open, chewing gum, unfortunately, makes you appear unrefined and coarse.

6. Use a fresh [unused] Kleenex tissue to blow your nose and discard it after each use.

   If with others, whether standing or sitting, unless it's impossible to do so, excuse yourself and step away from the others before you blow your nose.

   No matter where you are, be as unobtrusive as possible; therefore, do not dig...just dab. You are not mining for gold; you are merely blowing your nose.

   If more than basics are required, go to the washroom to carry out the task.

7. If, while amongst others, or even sitting at your desk, within earshot of others, you, accidently, burp or break wind [flatulence], do not act embarrassed or make a big scene; merely say, matter-of-factly, 'Excuse me," and continue with what you were doing.

8. If you find yourself going to sneeze, if you have time, turn and step away from those nearby, get out a Kleenex and sneeze into it. If there is not enough time for that, raise either one of your elbows and sneeze into the bend of your elbow.

   After you sneeze, merely say, matter-of-factly, 'Excuse me," and continue with what you were doing.

Lunchroom

1. If your employer provides a lunchroom, use it, if you plan to 'eat in'. Never eat at your workspace. It sends a message that you are 'backed up' and, therefore, cannot handle your assigned workload.

2. In spite of the fact you are on your own time, how you behave in the lunchroom will be noticed and judged by everyone. Act accordingly.

3. If you spill something, clean it up.

4. Use cutlery at all times, unless you are eating a sandwich, etc.

5. Hold cutlery as explained in the section on 'Cutlery'.

6. Chew with you mouth closed.

7. Do not chew and talk at the same time.

8. Use a serviette/napkin to wipe your hands.

9. If you used a tray to carry food to your table, always remove the food from the tray before you start to eat. Never consume the food directly from dishes sitting on the tray. Once the tray has been emptied, place it on its' end, on the floor, against the leg of your chair or place it on the designated tray stand.

10. Clean up after yourself, even if the company has someone assigned to maintain the area. Always leave the table clear and clean.

11. Be considerate of those who are sharing the lunchroom. Keep your voice down when conversing with those who are eating with you.

12. If a refrigerator is available, use it to keep your lunch cold, and safe to eat; but, do not abandon food. Make certain you throw out what you no longer want.

General

1. Smile!!! Maintain an up-beat demeanour. No one wants a sourpuss around them. How you appear to others will have a profound impact on promotions.

2. Speak at a normal volume, when addressing anyone. It is a good idea to ask a co-worker if your normal volume is too soft or too loud. Better they tell you than having everyone else thinking you are shy or obnoxious.

3. Do not pry into the lives of co-workers. If they wish for you to know, they will tell you. If they do not tell you, it is because they do not feel it is any of your business.

4. Share your personal happy events, at the right time [at lunch, etc.]; but, even then, keep it short, do not drag it out and do not keep repeating it. They will get it the first time and not appreciate it if you keep going over it.

5. Sharing happy events is one thing; bragging is wrong and will damage your image and permanently affect how others see you.

6. Follow what is written under 'Telephone'.

7. Be considerate of your co-workers. Take a moment to hold a door open for the person coming behind you, including when boarding an elevator.

8. Congratulate co-workers when they do something worthy of congratulations, be it within the work environment or in

their personal life. Congratulating someone is merely sharing their happiness and in no way detracts from you; in fact, if anything it will show others just what a warm and caring person you are.

Be sincere when complimenting or congratulating someone. If you do not mean it, the recipient, and those around them, will recognise that lack of sincerity and it will work against you.

Such actions will be weighed when a promotion is being considered. The fact that you know when, and how, to pay a compliment, will be important in deeming whether you would make a good Supervisor, Department Head, Vice-President or, even, President.

9. Do not 'suck up' to superiors, be they immediate supervisors or the company's Executive. Not only will they see right through you; but, so will your co-workers. Unless the superior is egotistical and vain, that type of pandering will not be respected and will, usually, be held against you.

10. Never gossip or bad-mouth anyone. When it comes to deciding the fitness of an employee for promotion, gossiping and bad-mouthing will definitely be considered a negative and will hold you back.

11. Do not waste your time or that of others. Respect your employer by providing a full day of work.

12. Respect other people's workspace.

13. If you need to stretch or take a break from your desk, do so....but do not bother others in the process. Walk to the

water cooler or out to the Reception or to the washroom; but, leave everyone else alone, so they can do their work.

14. Staying late, to impress the boss, usually does not work. All it does is to show everyone that you cannot get your work done within the allotted time frame as everyone else. Therefore, unless you have been requested to stay, or you have a very specific deadline that can only be accomplished by working overtime, don't stay.

15. Leave your personal problems at home. It will give you a break from them, which will be welcome; and, you will look at them differently after having a rest from dealing with them.

INTRODUCTIONS

N.B.   When being introduced, each situation must be analysed as to whether an handshake should be part of the introduction.

The rule has always been, if a gentleman is being introduced to a lady, unless the lady extends her hand, indicating she will accept an handshake, a gentleman should not extend his hand.

Certainly, in business, it is quite acceptable, and, indeed, proper to extend an hand to a woman who is also in business.

On the other hand, whether in business, or in a social situation, if the woman is an Orthodox Jew or strict Muslim, a gentleman should never offer his hand to shake.

Also, if the person, to whom you are being introduced, is holding food or drink, or anything else, do not offer to shake their hand unless they adjust the situation and offer you theirs.

In Your Home – up to six couples

Lead the individual or couple to the first couple or individual [always introduce couples together and singles on their own] to whom you are going to begin introductions [stand slightly to the side so the guests may clearly see and reach each other]; and, state, to the first individual or couple, 'Mary and George, I would like to introduce you to Helen and Peter Smith." Then turn to Helen and Peter and say, "Helen and Peter, I would like to introduce you to Mary and George Brown." In that way, each person's name is said twice. Make certain you speak clearly and are not in the way, so that they may shake each other's hand.

On occasion, you may find yourself not certain whether you should use first names [such as when people are not of the same social standing or age] during the introductions. In such a situation, always resort to, Dr. and Mrs. Humphries, I would like to introduce you to Margaret and Harold Sinclair." Then turn to the Sinclairs and say, "Helen and Peter, I would like to introduce you to Dr. and Mrs. Humphries." In using that approach, you leave it to the couple or individual being introduced with the more formal designation, to either leave it the way you have stated or to suggest that they call them by [and then they will tell them their first names].

Repeat the introduction process to all of the other guests.

In Your Home – more than six couples

More than six couples would most likely mean that you were not hosting a dinner party; however, even if you were [a buffet or backyard barbeque, etc] it is not necessary to attempt to introduce each arriving couple.

Take each couple or individual, after they have removed their coats, and introduce them to one or two couples whom you feel they would enjoy meeting. Conduct the introductions and then excuse yourself, so that you are available to greet the next arrivals or to 'circulate'.

Away From Home – By Yourself

As you extend you hand, to offer an handshake, say, 'How do you do, I'm _____ [use either your full name or just your first name, depending on the situation]'.

[Alternately]   As you extend you hand, to offer an handshake, say, 'Good morning [afternoon or evening], I'm _____ [use either your full name or just your first name, depending on the situation]'.

Following the other person reciprocating by giving their name and shaking your hand, respond by saying, 'It is very nice [or, 'it's a pleasure] to meet you.'

[When arriving for a meeting and you are speaking to a Receptionist]   'Good morning [afternoon or evening], I'm - _____ [use your full name]

Away From Home – With Your Spouse

'How do you do, we are Mary and Don Smith,

Or

'How do you do, this is my wife, Mary, and I'm Don Smith.

Away From Home – With Friends

Quite often, when out with friends, you run into others whom you know. Unless you are merely going to say 'hello' and keep moving, the correct action is to introduce those whom you have just met to those whom you are with. To do otherwise is to disregard the people you are with and act as if they are not with you.

Once you have completed the introductions, any ensuing conversation should be kept to a minimum, since you are taking time away from your original group.

Away From Home – With Friends – Adding To The Original Group

When you are out with a group of people, whether you are the host, the guest, or everyone is paying their own way, careful consideration should be given before you proceed to ask people whom you have just banged into, to join you.

How will those with whom you have been with, prior to meeting the new people, feel? Will they be a good match or will it produce an awkward situation?

Even asking the rest if they mind, places them in an awkward position.

Your first loyalty must be to the original group; therefore, approach the situation very judiciously. Possibly, pull one of the original group aside and ask them to be honest with how they feel about adding the others. Respect their opinion.

In Business – Introducing Yourself

[to a group] 'Good morning [afternoon, evening]; I'm John Smith, Vice-President of Gold Unlimited [or add 'of Toronto' if you feel they need that information.]
Or
[to one person] 'How do you do; I'm John Smith, Vice-President of Gold Unlimited [or add 'of Toronto' if you feel they need that information.]

In Business – Introducing One or More Plus Yourself

[to a large group or audience] 'I am [your name] [title if appropriate] and it gives me great pleasure to introduce the members of my group. First, I would like to introduce to you [then start with the highest ranking person] [use an open hand to indicate the person you are introducing, if there are more than one other besides yourself] Harry Brown, [title] of [company].

Continue to introduce each member of the group, with the name and title.

[to several] [first to the highest ranking] [you introduce the highest ranking in your party] 'Mr. Howell, I would like to introduce, John Smith, [Title] of [company]. Mr. Smith, this is Mr. Howell, [title] of [company]. Continue introducing John Smith to the one or two others. Once finished, introduce, one at a time of your group, allowing each to shake the hand of the others.

INVITATIONS

Extending An Invitation

An invitation, whether issued orally, via email, or printed and mailed, should contain all of the information you wish the guests to have and what the invitee requires to decide as to whether they will attend <u>and,</u> if attending, on what basis they will be attending.

Date & Time

Date and Time, plus any extra information the guest(s) should know in advance, so they may make an informed decision, is, obviously, vital information, necessary for the guests to determine their availability. Be specific by spelling both out completely. Never use a 12/10/10 format to indicate the date, since it could be misconstrued by the guest to mean either December 10th or October 12th.

When specifying the time, if it is a cocktail or 'drop-in' party, clearly state the hours of the party [5PM to 9PM]. For a dinner party, state: Cocktails at 7:00PM with Dinner at 8:00PM [or whatever times you determine]. The reason for doing that is very simple. You are informing your guests that you expect them to arrive at 7:00PM, enjoy a specified amount of time having cocktails [and hors d'oeuvre] [and to not gorge themselves on drinks and food] and then look forward to being served the meal at the stated time. Up front, it tells those who are habitually late in arriving that dinner will be served at the specified time; therefore, if they arrive considerably after 7:00PM [or whatever time is designated], they will only have the remaining time to have a cocktail, because you will be serving dinner when previously announced.

N.B. Guests who are late should never be afforded special treatment, especially at the expense of those who arrived on time. They are, quite simply, rude; giving little or no consideration for their host or fellow guests. Unless they have a valid excuse for the lateness, you should give serious consideration to dropping them from your future guests' lists. If you do not, they will quickly determine it is acceptable to arrive whenever they please.

Location

Always include in the invitation your full address, especially if it is the first time the invitees have been to your home. Provide street coordinates or other helpful information, especially if your location is the slightest bit difficult to find.

If you plan on hosting the party in your backyard, around your pool, or on your roof-deck, etc, include such information. By doing so, you are clear where it will be held; thus, you allow the invitee to accept or decline based on the complete situation. If it is summer and an invitee is allergic to mosquitoes, or being treated for an illness and must stay out of the sun, they will appreciate being told that you are planning an outdoor event, so they may either decline or bring repellent or dress appropriately. It also lets people know that they may like to bring a sweater or light coat/jacket in case the temperature drops.

Dress

Be clear on how you expect your guests to dress. If you are hosting a casual event, state that the dress will be casual. On the other hand, if you are hoping to have a slightly more 'dressy' affair, state 'gentlemen - jackets, please'. That should point out to all but the most socially inept, that you expect woman to also dress appropriately. The same holds true if you want your guests attired in 'gentlemen - suits, please' or 'gentlemen – tuxedos, please'.

If you inform your guests the event will be pool-side [or 'out on the patio' and they know you have a pool], be VERY specific as to whether you will be allowing your guests to use the pool. Can you imagine how upset you would be if you had planned a somewhat formal cocktail party on your patio and some of your guests, who know you have a pool, arrive in cover-ups and swimsuits? They would feel like clods, as would you.

The same holds true for any and all events; people appreciate being informed of your expectations, so they are appropriately attired.

Accepting An Invitation

Contrary to some advice, it is completely inexcusable not to respond to an invitation and just leave it to the host to guess whether you will attend.

Respond within a maximum of two to three days.

If it is a written invitation, and there is an enclosure card to be returned, complete it and mail it back.

Whatever method the hosts use to extend an invitation, be it mail, email, telephone or in person, is the method by which you should convey your intentions, unless the hosts have indicated an alternative method of responding.

Make certain you are clear when you communicate by stating exactly on behalf of whom you are accepting or declining.

[Example: "Harry and I, along with the three children, will be thrilled to attend."] In doing so, you clarify what is your understanding of the invitation. If the hosts did not mean for you to bring the children, or they did and you do not mention the children, it allows an opportunity to clarify.

N.B. Failure to respond, in a timely fashion, to an invitation, should warrant you being dropped from future invitations. It sends a message that you are not interested, even if you are.

ENTERTAINING AT HOME

Whether planning to 'order in' or have a 'formal' dinner party, formal cocktail party or swim/barbeque, the basic rules apply. Ultimately, following the correct rules of etiquette, each and every time you host an at-home event, will make it so much easier on your guests and yourself, since all the guess work is gone.

1. Invitations [See Invitations – page 89]

2. Planning the meal.

3. If extra dishes and cutlery are required, arrange for them as soon as possible. Order a few extra place settings plus extra dessert spoons and forks.

4. If extra glassware is being ordered, order more than just the bare number. [Appropriately sized plastic stemware and glasses are acceptable for use at events being held outdoors.] [If using glass stemware and glasses outside, be sure to have a dust pan and whisk close at hand in order to have any broken glass removed as quickly as possible.]

5. Make certain you have adequate table linens.

6. Is a disc jockey required? For inside or outside [different equipment might be required]? Book ASAP.

7. If you are hiring staff to assist, have them arrive at least thirty to forty-five minutes ahead of the party so you may provide them with full instructions as to your expectations and have them put any finishing touches to the event. Leave absolutely nothing to guessing.

8. Plan the liquor and wine requirements and assign someone to get it and set the date to do so [not the day of the party].

9. Determine how much ice will be required and assign someone to get it and set the time to do so [not on their way to the party].

10. If the party is being held outside, make certain you schedule the yard work for the day before.

11. If you have a swimming pool, schedule the pool to be cleaned the day before <u>and</u> skimmed again early on the morning of the party.

12. If it will be outdoors, inform your neighbours ahead of time and, on the day of the party, keep the volume of any music low enough so that it does not cause problems for your neighbours.

13. If you have pets, plan where they will be for the duration of the party. If it is a formal party, no animals should be present; no matter how sweet they are; because, they could damage the guests' attire.

14. The complete venue should be cleaned the day before.

15. Prepare the venue:
    - if parking will be a problem, offer suggestions in the invitation, such as 'courtesy Valet Parking will be available', or suggest public transit or taxis;
    - set table – sit-down or buffet [See Table Settings – page];
    - adjust [move] furniture, if necessary;
    - set-up washroom(s)

- an abundant supply of hand towels [an elegant, and yet inexpensive, alternative to paper guest towels is to buy a stack of washcloths or guest towels from IKEA or the $Store, roll each one and place them in a simple basket on the counter. If you do, make sure you place a large decorative basket or can nearby and toss one towel into it, so that your guests will get the message;

- flowers?

- liquid soap dispenser [a bar of soap causes a mess and is really gross] [Interesting point in history: President Dwight D. Eisenhower's wife, Mamie, insisted that each bar of soap in the White House be replaced with a fresh bar after being used, even in the washrooms where hundreds of guests attending State Dinners would be using the facilities.];

- a fresh roll of toilet paper [place several extra rolls in the vanity cabinet under the wash basin].

16. If it is an outdoor party, make certain there are a number of sand-filled-pails scattered around, to act as ashtrays. Otherwise, unfortunately, some will end up flicking their cigarette butts into your pool, grinding them out on your patio or grass, or over the fences into your neighbours' yards.

17. If it is an outdoor party, consider renting or buying several electric bug zappers and place them strategically around the patio and yard.

GREETING GUESTS TO YOUR HOME

Arrival of Guests – one to six couples

Hosts - Couple

Each guest should be greeted as they arrive by both hosts. After greeting each guest, the gentleman [if one of the hosts] should help them off with their coats and then place them on the bed in the bedroom nearest the door.

While the coats are being tended to, the other host should lead the guests to where the other guests are assembled and introduce them. [See Introductions – Page 83]

N.B. If the foyer is in close proximity to where the other guests are located [such as in a small apartment], hang the coats as you receive them; and, then immediately turn to the assembled guests and proceed to the introductions [See Introductions – Page 83].

The host taking care of the coats should listen carefully for the arrival of the next guests and the host conducting the introductions should do the same. If you are speaking with a guest, when you hear the knock or ring from the next arriving guests, excuse yourself and proceed to answer the door.

Host – Single

Each guest should be greeted by the Host and assisted with their coat. If there is a front hall closet, use it for the coats, in order to quickly process the coats. If you are going to place them on a bed, ask the guest(s) to wait while you take care of their coat; then, lead them to the other guests and introduce them [See Introductions – Page 83].

Arrival of Guests – more than six couples

When there are a large number of guests expected, there are two alternatives to correct greeting.

Either hire someone to act as a guest greeter [they can help serve the meal] or ask a friend if they would do the job, on your behalf, so that you are free to socialise with your guests.

Merely leaving the door un-attended for guests to wander in, find a place to hang their coats and then to find the bar, is a gauche faux pas and leaves your home open to strangers entering.

Whichever you choose to do, the person acting on your behalf should: answer the door; greet each person with a smile and a simple, "Good evening, may help you with your coat?" Once they have removed their coats, the greeter [if an employee] should then suggest that the guests proceed to the living room [or out on to the patio, or wherever is appropriate] where they will find 'Mr. & Mrs. Hosts' names, as well as the bar.

If a friend is acting as the greeter, they should do everything the same, except they should use the hosts' first name.

CONVERSATION PARTICIPATION

It is the responsibility of each and every guest to participate in conversations. You have been carefully selected because your Host(s) felt you would mix well with the others they selected and would contribute greatly to the wit or substance, or both, of the conversation. To do any less is to let down your Host(s), as well as yourself.

A good time may only be had by all, if everyone does their utmost to achieve the goal.

That said, do remember, participating is one thing; attempting to dominate and/or hijack the conversation is rude and may result in you being dropped from the Host(s) guest list.

SERVING DRINKS

Large Parties

When serving drinks, establish the pattern you wish to use, up front.

Is it to be self-serve, stationary bartender, roving bartender/server, stationary bartender/roving servers or hosts preparing and serving?

If you have hired a bartender, or someone has volunteered to act as bartender, the rules are the same:

1. Depending on the size of the party, the person in charge of the bar <u>should begin</u> to set up the bar anywhere from one hour for a large number, to thirty minutes for a small number, before the guests are scheduled to arrive.

2. Add ice to the tub or buckets where you will chill the beer and wine and then place the [assortment] beer and wine to chill.

3. Inspect each glass or stemware and polish, if necessary, as you set out the glassware in the appropriate place.

   - **Self-Serve:** in an orderly pattern on a table large enough to hold the entire bar requirements, including: glassware, ice, liquor, mix, wine and beer.

   - **Bar:** underneath or behind.

4. Place a stack of bar serviettes [napkins] either on the bar or next to the glassware and stemware display.

5. Fill a separate ice bucket and make certain there is a clean scoop [to be used <u>only</u> for ice] to use throughout the event.

6. If drinks are being served, make certain there are at least two clean trays for each server. One can be used to serve while the other is being loaded for the next service.

Small Parties

The bar should be set-up ahead of time, even if it is going to be a small gathering and the drinks are merely pre-prandial [pre-dinner]. Otherwise, there will be confusion in the kitchen as one person is attempting to get the drinks, while the other person is tending to the final touches for dinner.

<u>The host should determine ahead of time</u> as to whether they wish to:
- Serve just the first drink and let everyone help themselves to follow-up drinks;
- Serve each round, as you feel it is appropriate;
- Show each guest where the bar is and let them serve themselves.

Usually, pre-prandial cocktails are served for no longer than one hour prior to dinner being served. That length of time will, usually, mean that no more than two drinks will be consumed by your guests prior to going to the table for dinner and should allow you to control the volume of consumption.

[I once hosted a very formal dinner party at which two, very socially-prominent, couples insisted on consuming two large pitchers of martinis, in one hour, prior to dinner. They were well on their way to being blotto before we even arrived at the table. Planned and carried out, was a separate wine served at each of the seven courses, which was fine for the other four couples, plus us. Unfortunately, that was not the situation with the two couples who loved their martinis. By the end of the meal, they were so far gone that one of the, normally, very refined ladies was standing on her chair singing La Marseillaise. Not quite the after dinner entertainment I had planned.]

That time-frame should be followed even if hors d'oeuvres are being served. [If being served, the hors d'oeuvres should be started as soon as possible, so they will not conflict with guests being able to eat dinner.]

TABLE SETTINGS

Formal

1. Do not undertake a Formal Dinner if you do not either own, or plan to rent, the appropriate silver cutlery, crystal stemware and china. That is not meant as a snobby comment; it just means that you would be much more successful hosting a more casual meal.

2. Decide when first planning the event, whether you will be: 'plating' the courses, either from a serving cart in the dining room or in the kitchen; or, 'French Service' using Serving Staff.

3. If you plan on 'French Service', allow a minimum of at least twelve inches of space between each chair at the table, in order for Servers to be able to manoeuvre. [Servers should all wear white gloves.]

4. Food, whether plated or French Service, is always served from the left; and, dishes are always removed from the right.

5. Wine is always poured by the server standing on the right of each guest. Never does the server reach across a guest or the table.

6. Although well aware of the present popularity of 'chargers', I feel they are redundant and totally detract from your china and the set and decorated table. A confident host does not need to clutter their table with chargers. [If they are used, they must be removed at the same time the Main course plate is removed.]

7. Decide, when planning, which courses will be accompanied by wine. [See Food & Wine Matching – page 129]

8. Decide, when planning, which courses you will be having and in what order. Full 'Formal' dinner consists of:

    –   Amuse-Gueule [or sometimes called Amuse Bouche] [may be eaten with fingers, if in a small pastry cup or on a toast point; otherwise a small fork will be required]

    –   Appetiser – hot [soufflé] or chilled [pâté] etc. [small fork or small knife and fork if cutting is required] [Also see Asparagus – page 114]

    –   Soup – hot or chilled – use ½ cup serving [regular soup spoon for hot or a round soup spoon for chilled or creamed]

    –   Fish [fish knife and fork]

    –   Sorbet [usually a citrus flavour, meant to cleanse the palate] [small sorbet or tea spoon]

    –   Main [full-sized dinner knife and fork]

    –   Salad [meant to cleanse the palate] [salad fork] [no piece of salad should be so large as to require cutting]

    –   Cheese [individual cheese knife and fork]

– Sweet
[dessert spoon and dessert fork]

– Coffee and Tea
[tea spoon is placed on the saucer when served]

Remember when planning the menu, for a 'Formal' dinner, you must have enough cutlery to set each place at the table completely. It is simply not acceptable to wash cutlery between courses and then bring them back and put them back at each place.

Table Settings - Formal - Diagram

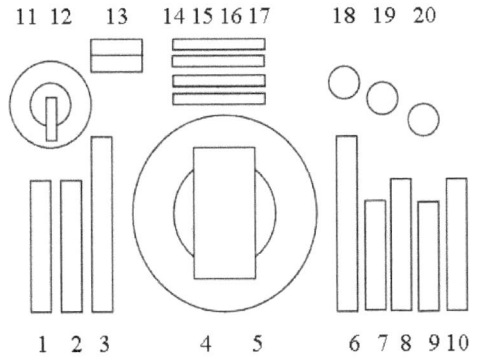

1. Appetiser Fork
2. Fish Fork
3. Dinner Fork
4. Dinner Plate
5. Linen Napkin
6. Dinner Knife
7. Sorbet Spoon
8. Fish Knife
9. Soup Spoon
10. Appetiser Knife
11. Bread/Butter Plate
12. Butter Knife
13. Place Card
14. Top-Cheese Knife
15. 2nd-Cheese Fork
16. Dessert Spoon
17. Dessert Fork
18. Water Goblet
19. Red Wine Goblet
20. White Wine Goblet

Table Settings – Others

All other table settings are based on the above 'Formal' table setting.

Positioning and content is exact; except, you would not have #13 and, most likely, you would have fewer courses, therefore, fewer pieces of cutlery. The cutlery you would have would be placed where they are in the formal setting.

Table Setting – Buffet

The only variant would be setting a 'Buffet' table.

Have the lay-out begin at the corner of the table closest to where the guest will enter the area.

Stack the plates as close to that corner as possible.

Leading from the plate stack, place the 'Main' hot dish, whether a roast, lasagne or oatmeal [breakfasts].

Next, the hot dishes that complement the 'Main'.

Leading around the table, following the hot dishes, should begin the cold dishes.

Just before the guest reach the end [where they started], should be the bread/rolls and butter, pickles, salt and pepper.

The very last thing should be a serviette/napkin rolled around a knife and fork.

That should have brought the guests back to where they entered, and they can leave the area without having to cross in front of those still queuing. [That is if you made the order of the food go in the correct direction.]

[If you live in an area where people cannot survive without a glass of ice tea in their hand, set up a station well away from the food table, preferably in the kitchen; this will prevent spillage and congestion around the food.]

Although tempting, NEVER put out your dessert(s), coffee and tea until the 'Main' table is finished....no matter what people demand.

When the guests are through with the 'Main' buffet, remove everything.

Set the dessert plate at the corner closest to the entrance, then the dessert(s) progressing along and around the table to the beverage area. If using thermos carafes, make certain you mark each so there is no confusion.

Place the dessert forks or spoons at the end of the line along with a fresh stack of serviettes/napkins.

Cup & Saucer / Teaspoon

The cup and saucer, plus the Tea Spoon, are never included in the original setting; but, appear after dessert, when coffee and tea is served.

Serviette / Napkin – Usage

The less handling the better; one, simply folded and placed on the dinner plate between 12 o'clock and 6 o'clock is total class.

Ones that have been folded in some fancy shape means they have been mauled by someone, most likely, with dirty hands.

Keep it sanitary; plus, make it easy for your guest to open, by merely folding them in half and then a three-fold.

[As a point of interest.....next time you are in a restaurant and they have some fancy serviette/napkin at your setting, it most likely was folded on top of some unsanitary surface by someone who had just finished cleaning the washrooms. Once again, less is more!]

[Also, when a Server or Maître d'Hôtel makes a big deal of grabbing your serviette/napkin, flipping it in the air and then trying to lay it across your lap: whether you realise it or not, he is mocking you because he does not feel you either moved fast enough to please him, or, you do not realise that you should place it on your lap. Either way, you should decline allowing him to place it on your lap by saying, 'Actually, I was not ready to touch my serviette/napkin; therefore, would you please bring me a fresh one that has not been waved around.]

Serviette / Napkin – Rings Usage

You will notice no serviette/napkin ring is shown. Napkin rings, for the most part, in today's world, are incorrectly used. Originally, the sole purpose of the ring was to identify which serviette/napkin belonged to which family member. A fresh linen serviette/napkin was placed at each place for Saturday dinner. When the meal was finished, each member of the family would place their personalised monogrammed silver ring over their gathered serviette/napkin and it would be saved in the sideboard and brought back out for each meal throughout the week. Guests would be not be supplied a ring, if they were only dining once with the family; however, if they were 'over-nighting', they would be given a unique ring, with its' own unique engraving, such as a rose, whereas another would have a daisy, etc. [That is why today's commercially sold sets offer four, six or eight different rings in the boxed assortment.] The servants would remember which guest was which flower and the correct ring could, therefore, be placed at the correct place for the remained of the week.

In today's world, we have, fortunately, reached a point where we are not so parsimonious when it comes to the use of serviettes/napkins. Whether linen or paper, a fresh one for each meal is correct; therefore, a ring is of no earthly use, unless of course one is attempting to make an impression.

Personally, I feel that, just as chargers detract from the beauty of a perfectly displayed table-top, so do serviette/napkin rings.

Certainly, less is more, when it comes to setting a proper <u>and</u> perfect table. Beautiful china, glistening crystal stemware, polished silver cutlery, crisp linen napery, fresh flowers, and elegant candlesticks with lighted candles.....what more could anyone ask for.....certainly not something as redundant as a charger or serviette/napkin ring!!!

Flowers

Fresh cut flowers elevate any table to 'special' and that is especially so when setting a 'formal', 'semi-formal', 'special' or 'party buffet' table. The display, or displays, depending on whether you plan to have one central arrangement with two candles/candelabra flanking, or one central candelabrum flanked by two identical arrangements, must be of an height as to not block the view across the table.

Either have the arrangements low enough to see over or tall enough to see under. Given most tables will not be large enough to handle high arrangements, having them lower is the practical way to handle the situation.

Napery – Table Linen / Placemats

Careful thought should be given to the table itself and to what you will be using to protect it or to hide it [if the table surface is not in good condition].

Will you be using a crisp white linen tablecloth or will you be using placemats? For a formal dinner, usually white linen tablecloth and serviette/napkins are the correct way to go. However, I often will use elegant hand-tatted placemats [crisp linen placemats can be used as an alternative] for a formal dinner, in order to show the beautiful wood-grained walnut dining-table surface. It really comes down to the look you are trying to achieve. [If you do opt to use placemats, they should be adequate in size to accommodate the entire place setting of cutlery and china. Goblets may sit off the placemat if necessary.

If using a tablecloth, many people will invest is a set of padded table-protectors [either readymade or custom made] which adds to the ambience by muffling the sounds of goblets, dishes and cutlery coming in contact with the table.

Seating Placement

Thoughtful and careful placement of your guests at the table will result in either an highly successful party or a disaster.

If there is a couple deemed to be the Guests of Honour, the female should be placed on the right-hand of the Host and the male on the right-hand of the Hostess.

Other couples should not, under normal circumstances, be placed next to one another. The exception would be if one of the two had special needs that were provided by the other.

Do your best to alternate male and female around the table; select who is next to whom, based on age, interests, etc.

Place Cards

Place cards are nice touch; but, it should be remembered they should be either hand-written or machine printed using a 'script font', so that they appear hand-written.

Grace

The Host(s) should determine <u>before</u> the beginning of the evening whether they plan to have a Grace said as soon as the guests are settled at the table and before and Toasts or Foodservice.

If it is to be said by a guest at the table, rather than the Host, the Host should ask if [Whoever] would please say the Grace.

If it to be said by the Host, the Host should merely ask if he may have a minute while he says Grace; and, then he should proceed.

Toasts

Offering <u>any</u> toast should be a sincere act, done properly.

At any banquet of formal dinner, whether the Queen is present or not, in countries with Her Majesty Queen Elizabeth II as Head of State, the correct procedure is, <u>before any food is served</u>, <u>the very first thing</u> should be to have whoever is going to deliver the opening toasts to rise and announce, 'Ladies and Gentlemen, would you all be upstanding, <u>raise your water glass</u> and join me in two toasts. First, to The Queen of [country's name], Her Majesty Elizabeth II. The Toaster then hoists their water glass and says, 'The Queen', to which everyone else raises their water glass and repeats, 'The Queen'.

Immediately, following that, the Toaster says, 'Also, please raise your glass to [country's name].' The Toaster then raises their glass, to the country's flag if it is nearby, and says, 'To [the country's name]', to which everyone else raises their water glass and repeats, 'To [country's name]'.

The Toaster then asks everyone to be seated and the food service may begin.

[Tradition dictates that the Queen and the country should always be toasted with water to show that they are sincere and sober people, who are aware of what they are saying.]

If it is a state dinner honouring another Head of State, Toasts are carried out much differently, including the timing and the use [usually] of Champagne or Wine.

N.B. During the Main Course, it is quite acceptable if one of the guests lightly clinks their wine glass with a clean spoon, in order to gain everyone's attention; and, then offer a Toast to the Host and Hostess.

Serviette & Napkin Usage

If you know for certain there will be a Toast prior to food service, you may leave your serviette/napkin on the dinner plate, until immediately after the Toast.

Either way, remove the serviette/napkin from the plate and unfold it until it is just doubled. Place it across your lap, with the double edge towards you.

Never tuck it in you shirt [if you are a man] or in the neck of your dress [if you are a woman].

When you wish to use it, take the right, top corner of the serviette/napkin, with your right hand [the reverse if left handed] and bring it to the right corner of your mouth. Dab it; then move it to the left corner; and then place it back on your lap with the fold, once again, towards you.

If, for any reason, you have to leave the table during dinner, dab the corners of your mouth and then excuse yourself to the lady on either side, then stand, place your serviette/napkin on your chair, and depart. When you return, merely pick up your serviette/napkin from the chair, retake your seat and place the serviette/napkin back onto your lap.

Your actions should be unobtrusive and as natural as possible, so that you do not disturb anyone else. As you pass by the Host or Hostess, merely say in a low voice, 'Please excuse me, I will only be a moment.' That way, they can decide to hold service of the next course, or to proceed.

Your serviette/napkin should remain on your lap until the Host or Hostess indicates the meal is finished. When you receive that instruction, slide your chair back, as you stand, place your serviette/napkin on the table directly in front of you, step away from your chair and slide it partially back under the table, if it is making passage difficult; otherwise leave the chair.

Order of Guests Served

Whether the food is being served using French Service [a white-gloved Server, standing to the left of the dinner guest, serves each course's item(s) of food from a silver tray and places them onto the dinner plate of the guest, in a pre-planned placement] or it is being plated in the kitchen or at a serving table in the dining room, there is a precise order in which the guests must be served.

The female 'Guest of Honour' is the first to be served, followed by the male 'Guest of Honour'; next, the oldest female; then the next oldest and finally the youngest female; next would be the oldest gentleman, next oldest, down to the youngest.

The second last person to be served is the Hostess; and, the Host is always the last.

Accepting & Declining Food

If the meal is being French Served, when the Server asks if you would like [whatever], merely smile and say, 'Yes, thank you' or 'No thank you.' No further comments are expect or required.

On the other hand, if the food is being passed, and you do not wish to have any of a particular item, merely accept the bowl or platter when it is passed to you and then pass it on to the next person to your left. Making a comment about not liking it, or that you are allergic to it, etc, is not appropriate.

If the meal is being plated, whether in the kitchen or at tableside, accept the plate as presented and merely leave the item you do not wish to consume, untouched, on your plate. Do not 'play' with it or attempt to hide it under a pile of bones.

Say absolutely nothing, unless asked. If asked, simply state, 'Regretfully, I'm allergic to that; but, I made up for it with the rest of the delicious meal,' or, 'I'm not too fond of [whatever]; but, I made up for it with the rest of the delicious meal.'

Food Tip

Over your lifetime, hopefully, you will be offered food that is unknown to you, whether because it is ethnic in origin; or, it contains something to which you have not been exposed.

By taking advantage of those opportunities, you may just be surprised at how many food items you actually learn to enjoy. Also, I can assure you, as you get older, your taste buds really do change. Quite often, food that you could not stand when you were young becomes a favourite later on. Many times it turns out that it was just the way something was cooked that resulted in turning you off.

So, do yourself a favour; continually allow yourself to try new dishes and new food items.

When To Begin To Eat

Unless the Hostess, or if there is no Hostess, the Host bids you to proceed to eat, <u>it is absolutely not acceptable to begin to eat until the Hostess [or Host] begins</u>.

By following the Host's lead, you also save yourself the embarrassment of using the wrong utensil, should you be unsure which is correct.

[When young, my parents were hosting a dinner party in honour of a well-known woman who had spent much of her life working in Africa building small medical clinics to help the indigenous people. It was tacitly expected for each attending couple to make a sizable contribution to her efforts near the evening's end. Being the 'Guest of Honour' she was served first for each course and, then, would proceed to consume that course, without waiting for everyone else. Realising that she might be embarrassed if she noted others waiting. Mother merely nodded to each guest, as they were served, to proceed. When the Main Course was served, it consisted of roast beef, duchess potatoes and minted baby peas. The 'Guest of Honour', upon receipt of her plate, took her knife, mixed the peas in with the potato, and then lifted the mixture to her mouth using her knife. Without missing a beat, Mother merely indicated to the next lady being served to do the same thing. The balance of the table followed as if it was de rigueur.]

My purpose in relating that incident is to point out that it is the duty of the Host and Hostess to always ensure your guests are never embarrassed or made to feel awkward or unwelcome. The Host and Hostess should lead by example. In the above situation, it was much more important to make the Guest of Honour feel comfortable and welcome, than following protocol.

Ultimately, etiquette is all about being mannerly toward others.

Bread & Rolls – Correct Eating Method

Bread, no matter in what form, should be placed on your bread and butter plate, which you will find located above, slightly to the left, of your fork(s). There should be a small butter knife placed on the plate.

If a Server offers you a roll or a piece of bread, merely say, 'Yes, thank you' or 'No, thank you'. If there is a selection of various grains or types, merely tell them what you would like to have and leave it up to them to place it on your bread and butter plate.

The butter may be served in small cuts or balls, by the Server or it may be placed in one or more areas around the table. If served, respond in the same manner as you would for the bread.

Should the bread/rolls and butter be placed on the table, for self-serving, leave it until the Main Course. Once the main Course has been served and eating has begun, it is quite proper to either pick up the bread/rolls basket, if it is in front of you, or, to ask if the guest sitting closest to the basket would begin the bread being passed.

If, indeed, you are the one who is initiating the passing, you should lift the basket, and while still holding it, turn to your right and offer it to the person on your right, by saying, 'Do you care for some bread/roll?' If they say that they would, merely let them take one and then help yourself to a piece of bread or a roll, place it on your bread and butter plate, and then, turning to your left, say, 'Would you care for some bread/roll?' If they says, yes, respond with, 'May I hold the basket for you?' Once they have taken a piece of bread or a roll, merely say, 'Would you please pass this.'

Repeat the exact same process for the butter, making certain you firmly hold it whilst the lady on your right, using the butter knife accompanying the butter dish, takes the butter from the butter dish you are holding. The butter should be placed on the bread and butter plate, beside the piece of bread/roll. Only take enough butter for the one piece of bread/roll that you have on your plate. Never use your butter knife to take butter from the main butter dish.

When you desire a piece of bread or roll, using the thumb and forefinger of your left hand, break off a small piece, the size of one bite, while holding it over the bread and butter plate with the thumb and forefinger of your right hand. Then lay the remainder of the bread back on the plate. With your right hand pick up the butter knife from the bread and butter plate and use it to take a small dab of butter from the amount you have previously placed on the bread and butter plate. Next, place the butter on the small piece of bread or roll that you are holding in your left hand; but, do not slather it all over. Place the butter knife back on to your bread and butter plate, with your right hand, and then place the piece of bread into your mouth using your left hand.

- Never use your butter knife to cut your bread or roll. Always break off one piece at a time.
- Never break off a large piece of bread.
- Never spread the entire piece of bread at once or cut the roll in half and spread the halves with butter.
- Always, just break off one small piece at a time and eat it before you start another piece. The piece should be small enough for you to be able to chew and swallow quickly, in case you have to respond to the conversation from either of your seat-mates.

Passing Items

Unless there are individual salt and pepper meant for just you, all items placed in front of your position at the table are your responsibility to pass. Depending on the formality of the dinner, that could be: gravy; salt and pepper; sauces; cranberries; pickles; mustard; bread/rolls; butter; bowls and/or platters of food.

Initiate the passing by lifting the item, and while still holding it, turn to your right and offer it to the person on your right, by saying, 'Do you care for some [whatever]?' If they say that they would, merely let them take one and then help yourself to [whatever], and then, turning to your left, say, 'Would you care for some [whatever]?' If they says, yes, say, [if appropriate] 'May I hold [whatever] for you?' Otherwise, merely say, 'Would you please pass this.'

121

Removing Something From Your Mouth

Contrary to what many do, if you find yourself with something in your mouth that you wish to remove, whether it is a bone or food that you do not wish to consume, do not spit it into your serviette/napkin [the last thing you want is to have a wad of food wrapped in your serviette/napkin, sitting on your lap, for the rest of the meal.

Be as unobtrusive as possible and merely remove it with your thumb and first two fingers and place it on the side of your dinner plate. Wipe your fingers on your serviette/napkin and then continue to eat.

Asparagus – Correct Eating Method

When asparagus is served as an appetiser or a vegetable as part of the main course, whether hot or chilled, it should always be eaten by picking it up with ones' finger, at the cut end.

Dip the free end into an accompanying small dish of Hollandaise and repeat until the spear has been consumed. Place the small piece of the spear that you held back onto the plate and proceed to do the same with each spear.

If the asparagus is served, in the true classic fashion, accompanied by a soft-boiled egg, use the small egg-spoon, which should be on the saucer, next to the soft-boiled egg (nesting in an eggcup, top-cracked but unopened); hold the egg with your left hand; slide the tip of the spoon into the crack near the top of the egg and lift off the cap. Using the spoon, scoop out the white of the egg in the cap and eat it. Next, pick-up the first spear by the cut end and dip the tip of the spear into the yolk of the soft-boiled egg and then eat that portion. Repeat until the spear is eaten to where it is being held, then place the small remaining piece back onto the plate. Continue until you have eaten all of the spears.

Once you have finished the asparagus, it is quite permissible if you use the egg spoon to finish eating the balance of the soft-boiled egg.

Spareribs – Correct Eating Method

Although highly doubtful an Host would serve spareribs at a Formal Dinner, they very well might be served at a regular dinner party; therefore, it is helpful to know the correct method to use to eat them, should you not wish to use your fingers.

Using you knife to hold the rack, use your knife to sever a block of three to four ribs from the main rack; using your knife and fork, turn the newly severed block of ribs over.

While holding the smaller block of ribs with your fork, use your knife to run along the right-most edge of the right-most rib and pry the meat from the bone as you go. As you do, slide the knife slightly under the right edge of the length of the rib.

Repeat the technique along the left-side of that rib. Once the entire length of the rib has been completed, you should be able to lift the rib away from the meat, using your knife and fork to place the rib to the side of your plate.

Eat the newly detached meat; then repeat the process with the next rib.

After just a few ribs, you will be quite amazed at how easy the process is and how quickly you can 'clean the bones' much better than you ever did cutting them apart and eating them with your fingers.

Of course, it also leaves you with clean hands, just in case fingerbowls are not supplied.

Fingerbowl Usage

Usually, the only time a fingerbowl is used, nowadays, would be following a course that involved using your fingers to convey food to your mouth, such as asparagus, corn-on-the-cob or spare ribs [see Asparagus – page 114 and Spare Ribs – page 114].

The bowl, set on a saucer, would be placed in front of you, following the removal of the plate for that course. In the bowl should be warm water and a slice of lemon.

Dip your fingertips into the warm water and rub the lemon discreetly between them to remove and grease or sauce. Dry your fingertips on your serviette/napkin. If you feel your lips are greasy, take the dampened portion of your serviette/napkin which you just used to dry your fingertips and, using one hand, discreetly dab your lips with the dampened serviette/napkin. Never dip the serviette/napkin into the fingerbowl in order to moisten it.

Posture

Correct posture at the dinner table, whether a formal dinner or just dining with the family, is vitally important.

<u>NEVER</u>, **<u>EVER</u>** place your elbows on the table. It is the singular worst faux pas one can make while sitting at the dinner table and is an insult to the Host(ess) and all other at the table.

Slouching indicates you are bore and not the least bit interested in the meal and the accompanying conversation. Even if that is the situation, you have accepted the invitation to dine at the table, so the least you can do is to act interested and sit up straight.

When not eating, or in between courses, simply place your hands in your lap and never fidget with cutlery or other table items; again it sends a message that you are bored.

If you are that bored, either make an effort to stimulate the conversation by contributing to it; or, excuse yourself and forego the meal.

Sitting at the table and insulting the other dinners, showing boredom, is not an acceptable alternative.

CUTLERY

General Usage

It is safe to say, nothing demonstrates ones level of etiquette grooming as does how one holds their cutlery.

Prior to cutlery, people ate with their hands. They tore apart joints of meat; scooped vegetables with their hands and spit unwanted food and bones onto the floor, for the wandering dogs to consume. Times have changed; but, unfortunately, some people still eat as though cutlery has yet to be invented. If it isn't in a bun, they are lost as to how to eat it.

As with many aspects of etiquette, those who dismiss the importance of correct cutlery handling, do so at their peril; because, they will never be accepted socially.

During a recent conversation with several highly respected Barristers, they mentioned how surprised they were to have noticed several of their peers were in desperate need of being instructed in the correct way to hold their cutlery. They felt badly for them, since something that is so public and obvious may have a profound impact on how others see and treat them professionally.

Each piece of cutlery has been refined, over hundreds of years, to be used in very specific ways. When they are used contrary to how they were intended, it will appear, at the least, to be very awkward and at the most, the person is a **Clod**.

Ultimately, each piece of cutlery's only function is to convey food from the plate to the diner's mouth; and, to do it without soiling ones hands.

Many people in Europe and Canada place the cutlery at the place setting with the tines of the forks curved down and the spoons with the bowls facing the tabletop. In fact most European-made silver is manufactured with the 'hallmarks' on the opposite sides of the cutlery, to what is 'the norm' in the USA.

The reason is quite simple. Once the knife and fork are picked up, they are not set back down until the diner has finished with that course.

The complete opposite, for the most part, in the USA; where, for some reason, over the years, they have developed the habit of cutting a piece of meat or vegetable, laying the knife down on the plate, passing the fork to their right hand, skewering whatever they just cut, moving it to their mouth, moving the fork back to their left hand, picking up the knife with their left hand and, then, do it again with the next piece. Whew!!! I am worn out. What a tedious and inefficient way to convey food to ones mouth.

Believe me when I state, I am not making fun of how it is done; I am merely pointing out that it is inefficient and, actually, quite difficult.

For instance, when something is difficult to skewer or move up onto the fork tines, with that method, one must use either a piece of bread in their other hand, or the fingers of the free hand, to push the food onto the fork.

Not only will the food, most likely be cold, by the time one finishes; but, ones hands are food-caked and greasy.

Using the European and Canadian method, one merely: skewers the piece of what they wish to eat, with their fork, in their left hand; holds it in place while they cut it loose with their knife; then lifts the fork, with the piece of food still skewered, to their mouth; and, then repeat the process. If sauce needs to be placed on the skewered item, one merely pushes some onto the piece of food with the knife.

The fork is never, ever, turned over to be used as a shovel. Food is either skewered by the fork or it is pushed onto the outer-curve-side of the fork and then conveyed to the mouth. Using this method, even peas would be moved from the plate to the diner's mouth. That is why the fork of European cutlery is curved more than American made forks.

This simple and effective way to convey food is followed whether using an 'Appetiser' Knife and Fork, 'Main' Dinner Knife and Fork, 'Cheese' Knife and Fork, 'Fruit' Knife and Fork, 'Dessert' Knife and Fork or a 'Dessert' Fork and Spoon.

Cutlery Placement – When Pausing

If you wish to pause, while eating, whether or not you are leaving the table, NEVER place your cutlery back onto the table surface, even if there are rests for the cutlery.

Place the left hand item, on the dish, from the centre out to 8 o'clock and the right hand item, on the dish, from the centre out to 4 o'clock. That is a signal that you are not finished.

Cutlery Placement – When Finished

When one has finished eating a particular course, place the cutlery used during that course [if two implements, place them together, side by side, as they left your hands] at the 'four o'clock' position of the plate or in the rimmed soup [if there is an accompanying saucer, do not place the cutlery on the saucer].

129

Cutlery - Holding

Knife

Grasp the knife in your right hand [all instructions should be reversed if left-handed], between your thumb and index [first] finger; curl your fingers [other than thumb] around the shaft of the knife; extend your index finger and place in on the shaft; as you cut, press down with your index finger. Do not saw back and forth. Press down and slightly move the knife back and forth. The end of the knife handle should not extend beyond your hand.

Fork

Grasp the fork in your left hand, with the tines curving down, between your thumb and index [first] finger; curl your fingers [other than thumb] around the shaft of the fork; extend your index finger and place in on the shaft. The end of the fork handle should not extend beyond your hand.

N. B. There will be times when you are served courses that require you to use a knife and fork, other than for the Main course, such as:

Appetiser course – typical in shape but smaller than normal and are held and used in the normal manner;

Cheese course – typical in shape but smaller than normal and are held and used in the normal manner;

Dessert course – typical in shape but smaller than normal and are held and used in the normal manner;

Fish course – the knife is an unusual shape and the fork looks somewhat like a dessert fork and are both held and used in the normal manner.

Soufflé course – may be served with either a knife and fork combination that is similar to a dessert knife and fork; <u>or</u>, a spoon and fork combination that is similar to a dessert spoon and fork.

Salad course – no salad should ever be served that requires any portion of it to be cut. All pieces should be mouth-sized to begin with; therefore, if properly served, all that would be used would be a salad fork, which is similar in size to a dessert fork. It may be used in ones right hand or left hand, whether the user is right or left handed. When finished, the fork is placed at the 4 o'clock position.

Spoon – Soup

With your right palm facing up, place the spoon end under your thumb where it meets the rest of your hand, bowl-side up, and the shaft between your index and second finger.

Move the spoon from the centre of the soup bowl towards the 12 o'clock position of the bowl; and then, move the soup spoon to your mouth.

Tilt the side of the spoon against your lips and allow the liquid to enter your mouth. Do not slurp the liquid or turn the spoon and thrust the bowl into your mouth.

Once the spoon is empty, repeat the steps until the bowl has been emptied. As you reach the bottom, it is permissible to slightly tilt the bowl; **but**, <u>it must be tilted away from you</u>, NEVER towards you.

When finished, place the soup spoon between the centre of the bowl and 4 o'clock.

Spoon – Dessert

Whether the dessert spoon is being used in combination with a dessert fork [the correct method] or by itself, the spoon is held with your right palm facing up, place the spoon end under your thumb where it meets the rest of your hand, bowl-side up, and the shaft between your index and second finger.

When used with a dessert fork, the fork holds the dessert while the dessert spoon is used to cut or break one piece away from the rest.

Once separated, determine whether the spoon should be used to hold the piece while the fork skewers the piece and conveys it to the mouth or the fork is used to push the piece of dessert onto the spoon and then conveyed to the mouth.

Whether a lone dessert spoon or a dessert fork and spoon, when finished the cutlery should be placed at the traditional 4 o'clock position, indicating you a finished.

Spoon – Sauce/Gravy

Although rarely used, a Sauce Spoon, looks like a cross between a Dessert Spoon and a Fish Knife; with a flat side, the length of the bowl and a curved side on the opposite.

Merely hold the spoon in the standard way and slide it across the plate or dish, collecting the sauce or gravy. Bring it to your lips; sip it from the spoon; then repeat until finished.

Spoon – Sorbet

If a sorbet is served between the Fish and Main courses, hold the spoon [which is almost like a Teaspoon] in the usual way; take small scoops of the sorbet, from closest to you and then work further and further away, until finished.

Place the spoon on the accompanying saucer, on the right side of the stemmed pedestal.

STEMWARE – HOW TO HOLD & USE

Stemware should be chosen so that it 'elevates' the linear look the china and cutlery provides and really brings the table alive. Make certain the pattern lifts rather than flattens the over-all 'look'. To do that, either get a chair and sit to view it with your china and cutlery or stoop so that you are looking at it from roughly the same level as your head will be when sitting at your dinner table. If you do this, prior to purchase, I guarantee you will select a different pattern than you would have, had you just stood there looking at it.

Usually, you should select a Water, Red Wine and White Wine Goblet, as well as Old Fashion and Tumbler, in your pattern.

The dining table stemware of Water, Red and White Wine Goblets, **NEVER** should be used in the living room or anywhere but on the dining room table.

The reverse is true of your Old Fashion and Tumbler which are meant for pre-prandial drinks. By using them for drinks before dinner, it is a way of 'inviting' your guests to your table. The Old Fashion is used for any drink being served 'neat' or 'on the rocks'. Use the Tumbler for any mixed drink.

If wine is to be served before dinner, have separate wine goblets [Riedel Vitis is a beautiful and comfortable goblet that is perfect with any decor].

At your table, offer both chilled 'still' and 'effervescent' and avoid using ice cubes [they cause sweating of the glass, which can lead to dripping and slipping; as well as causing splashing if they suddenly slip while the person is drinking].

When filling <u>any</u> wine goblet, it should only be filled to $1/5^{th}$ of the goblet. Remember, wine is to accompany the meal, not become a course unto itself. This is especially true if you are serving a different wine with each course.

If you are going to be re-using either the white or red goblet for a different course's wine, have a pitcher of fresh tap water on your sideboard, along with an empty bowl. Merely take each glass to the sideboard, pour a small amount of water into it, swirl it around several times, empty the water into the bowl and return the glass to the appropriate dinner guest. Once you have completed doing it for everyone, proceed to pour the next wine.

When you are completely through with that particular glass, it should be removed.

Hold stemware mid-way up the stem. Do not hold any wine glass by its' pedestal, unless you are judging a competition; to do so is pretentious and will cause you embarrassment.

COFFEE & TEA SERVICE

After dinner Coffee & Tea may be served at either the dining room table or in the living room; and, is the prerogative of the Hostess where.

Brought to the Hostess and placed at either her place at the dining room table or placed on a small table adjacent to where she is sitting in the living room, should be a silver tray, large enough to hold one each: coffee pot; tea pot; creamer; milk jug; sugar pot; and, a cup and saucer for each guest and a similar number of teaspoons.

Using the same serving pattern as for the food, the Hostess asks the first person to be served if they would prefer coffee or tea.

Once they respond, the Hostess should then ask how they take their coffee or tea.

If sugar is requested, the Hostess places the requested amount of sugar into the empty cup, followed by either cream, for coffee, or milk, for tea. NEVER should cream be used in tea [the butter fat changes the flavour of the tea]; finally, the coffee or tea is poured into the cup, a teaspoon is placed on the right-hand side of the saucer and, then, the Hostess passes the cup and saucer to the correct person. [She should hand it to the person on either her left or right and ask them to pass it – then they repeat the action until it reaches the intended guest.]

The Hostess continues this until she is the last to be served; then, she serves herself.

PORT & LIQUEUR SERVICE

While the Hostess is serving the coffee and tea, it is the perfect time for the Host to offer Port and Liqueurs to the guest, whether still at the dining room table or in the living room.

The same serving order used for the food and coffee and tea service, should be used to serve the Port and Liqueurs.

FOOD & WINE MATCHING

Here is a basic wine and food matching chart to get you started. This is just a basic list in terms of the wines or dishes; by experimenting, you will discover many surprising matches.

NOTE:

New World includes regions and countries such as California, Australia, New Zealand, Chile, Argentina, Canada, South Africa, New York, Oregon and Washington, among others.

Old World includes France, Germany, Spain, and Italy.

Start with a Dish

Salads: Sauvignon Blanc, Riesling, Pinot Blanc, Pinot Gris, Pinot Grigio, Un-oaked Chardonnay, Sparkling Wine, Champagne, Gamay, New World Pinot Noir

Casserole/Shepherd's Pie: New World Chardonnay, New World Cabernet Sauvignon, Zinfandel, Syrah

Chicken (Cream Sauce): Sauvignon Blanc, Sparkling Wine, Champagne, Un-oaked Chardonnay, Riesling, Pinot Blanc, Pinot Gris, Pinot Grigio

Chicken (Grilled): Riesling, Shiraz, Syrah, Zinfandel

Chicken (Lemon or Citrus): Riesling, Chablis, Un-oaked Chardonnay

Chilli: Riesling, Zinfandel, Shiraz

Foie Gras: Sauternes, Icewine, Tokaji

Game (Venison, Duck, Pheasant, Quail, Rabbit, Boar) and Turkey: New World Chardonnay, Pinot Noir, Shiraz, Syrah, Rioja

Lamb: Bordeaux, Rioja, Syrah

Pasta/Pizza/Lasagna/Cannelloni/Ratatouille/Spaghetti:
Riesling, Sangiovese, Chianti, Montepulciano d'Abruzzo, Primitivo, Barbaresco

Pork (Spicy): Gewurztraminer, Un-oaked Chardonnay, Off-Dry Riesling, Sauvignon Blanc, Dolcetto, Chianti

Pork (Grilled or Plain): New World Chardonnay, New World Pinot Noir, Zinfandel

Red Meats (Spicy): Gamay, Pinot Noir, Red Burgundy

Red Meats (Rich: Osso Bucco, Beef Bourguignonne): Oaked Chardonnay, Cabernet Sauvignon, Shiraz, Syrah, Dolcetto, Pinot Noir, Barolo

Red Meats (Grilled): Sauvignon Blanc, Sangiovese, Chianti, Zinfandel, Primitivo

Seafood/Shellfish (Grilled/Smoked): Un-oaked Chardonnay, Sauvignon Blanc, Pinot Noir

Seafood/Shellfish (Butter or Cream Sauce): Oaked Chardonnay, Chablis, Sparkling Wine, Champagne

Spicy/Asian Dishes/Sushi: Gewurztraminer, New World Chardonnay, Off-Dry Riesling, Sauvignon Blanc

Vegetables/Eggs/Quiche: Sauvignon Blanc, Sparkling Wine, Un-oaked Chardonnay, Riesling, Pinot Blanc, Pinot Gris, Pinot Grigio

Cheese (Blue, Stilton): Tawny Port, Vintage Port, Sauternes, Madeira

Cheese (Goat): Sauvignon Blanc, Sparkling Wine, Champagne, Cabernet Franc

Cheese (Creamy: Brie, Camembert): Sauvignon Blanc, Sparkling Wine, Champagne, Un-oaked Chardonnay, Riesling, Pinot Blanc, Pinot Gris, Pinot Grigio

Desserts (Fruit Flan, Lemon Cake, Citrus-Based Desserts): Icewine, Sauternes, Late Harvest Wines, Tokaji

Dessert (Crème Brulee, Sorbet, Ice Cream): Icewine, Sauternes, Tawny Port, Late Harvest Wines, Cream Sherry, Moscato D'Asti

Dessert (Chocolate): Framboise, Strawberry Liqueur, Raspberry Liqueur, Tawny Port, Sauternes

Nuts: Tawny Port, Madeira, Cream Sherry

Start with Wine

White Wines

Chardonnay: seafood with butter sauce, chicken, pasta with cream sauce, veal, turkey, ham, Emmenthal, Gruyeres, Port-Salut

Riesling: mild cheese, clams, mussels, Asian dishes, sashimi, ham, pork, lobster Newberg, Tandoori chicken, Coquilles St Jacques

Sauvignon Blanc: oysters, grilled or poached salmon, seafood salad, Irish stew, ham, chevre, goat cheese and strongly flavored cheeses, asparagus quiche

Gewurztraminer: spicy dishes, Thai food, curry, smoked salmon, pork and sauerkraut, Muenster, spiced/peppered cheeses, onion tart

Red Wines

Cabernet Sauvignon: duck, spicy beef, pate, rabbit, roasts, spicy poultry, cheddar, blue cheese, sausage, kidneys

Pinot Noir: braised chicken, cold duck, rabbit, charcuterie, partridge, roasted turkey, roasted beef, lamb, veal, truffles, Gruyeres

Merlot: braised chicken, cold duck, roasted turkey, roasted beef, lamb, veal, stew, liver, venison, meat casseroles

Shiraz: braised chicken, chili, goose, meat stew, peppercorn steak, barbequed meat, spicy meats, garlic casserole, ratatouille

WHICH WINE WITH WHICH SPICE?

White Wines

Chardonnay	• Cinnamon • Garlic • Marjoram • Rosemary • Saffron • Tarragon • Thyme
Pinot Blanc	• Chives • Garlic • Oregano • Parsley • Thyme
Pinot Gris	• Basil • Fennel • Saffron • Tarragon • Thyme
Riesling	• Capers • Caraway • Dill • Chives • Ginger • Sage
Sauvignon Blanc	• Coriander • Ginger • Lemongrass • Parsley • Green Pepper

Red Wines

Cabernet Franc	<ul><li>Basil</li><li>Bay Leaf</li><li>Rosemary</li><li>Savoury</li><li>Thyme</li></ul>
Cabernet Sauvignon	<ul><li>Bay Leaf</li><li>Rosemary</li><li>Sage</li><li>Tarragon</li><li>Thyme</li></ul>
Gamay	<ul><li>Basil</li><li>Oregano</li><li>Sage</li><li>White Pepper</li></ul>
Merlot	<ul><li>Bay Leaf</li><li>Garlic</li><li>Juniper</li><li>Rosemary</li><li>Sage</li><li>Thyme</li></ul>
Pinot Noir	<ul><li>Basil</li><li>Chervil</li><li>Mint</li><li>Thyme</li></ul>
Zinfandel	<ul><li>Basil</li><li>Bay Leaf</li><li>Black Pepper</li><li>Mild Chilli</li><li>Oregano</li><li>Paprika</li></ul>

ENTERTAINING AWAY FROM HOME

Personal

Many people today have concluded that, with their busy schedules and smaller apartments, condos or homes, it is better for them to reciprocate social obligations by entertaining away from their home.

It can even be cost effective; but, only if you are cautious in your planning. The biggest difference between entertaining at home and at an away-from-home facility is the liquor costs. At home, although you, as the host, will be expected to provide the mixes and some of the liquor, most thoughtful guests will bring at least one bottle of wine, or a case of beer, or a bottle of their favourite liquor. In a commercial facility, no liquor from the outside is legally allowed. Thus, unless you have extraordinary friends who will 'kick in' towards the cost of the liquor, your bill for the liquor portion of the bill could be very high.

One way around out-of-control liquor costs is to establish the parameters at the time you issue the invitations.

You will remember, in the section on 'Invitations', I state that you should be very clear about all facets of the invitations, so those whom you invite may be able to base their decision to accept or decline, based on all of the conditions.

By stating that dinner [or hors d'oeuvres, snacks or whatever food you decide], along with wine [and beer if you feel you can afford that] will be provided. Any liquor consumed will be the responsibility of the person ordering.

In that way, no one will be surprised if they accept and attend. You, in turn, will be able to establish ahead of time, working with the facility, exactly how many bottles of wine [and beer if you are including that] you will be willing to accept on your bill.

TIP Before the event starts, have the facility set the number of wine bottles aside [both red and white] of the brand you have decided to use. [Usually, the best buy is the 'House' wine; because, they don't want an unpleasant wine to have their business' name attached to it and they want to demonstrate how affordable their place is.] Once they are separated, initial each bottle and tell them you will only pay for initialed bottles, at the end of the evening.

Every so often, go by the bar and check to see how many have already been finished and check to see the others are still there and unopened. If you have any question, such as a bottle is missing, immediately speak to management.

If all of the initialled bottles are consumed before the end, it then is the facility's responsibility to ask you if you wish to add more to the bill. If you do, initial the additional bottles. Never initial a bottle that is already open.

Also, up-front, establish how much TIP the restaurant will be charging when you negotiate the terms for food and wine, etc. If they attempt to change it, refuse to pay the difference.

Arrivals & Departures

As the host, you should be at the facility at least thirty minutes prior to the scheduled time for arrival.

Check where you are being placed. [If available, a separate room can really work to your advantage because you can be more boisterous and monitor the wine and beer distribution must better.]

Make certain they have set for the correct number of guests and that the servers assigned to your group are clear on what you have ordered and expect.

Greet each guest as they arrive and show them where to hang their coat.

Remind them of the way the bar will be working and show them where they should go to use it [there might be a special spot at the bar for your group].

Attempt to introduce each newly arrived guest to at least one other guest, so they are not left standing by themselves, when you go to greet the next arrivals.

Unless you absolutely feel compelled to do so, DO NOT use name badges. They are tacky and make most people feel as if they are back in school.

Whenever the food service was scheduled to be served, make certain a few minutes prior to the established serving time that management is ready to proceed. Check as it proceeds that all of your guests are receiving what they should.

Above all, remember you are the host.

As the evening progresses, keep an eye on your guests, as you mingle, and make certain you say 'goodnight' to each and every guest.

Do not take time from your guests to settle the bill; settle it after everyone has departed.

DATING

Please note: The following is applicable to dates whether opposite sex or same sex.

The Invitation / Who Is The Host

Transportation / Venue Protocol

Although you will hear that the rules for dating have changed, don't believe it.

Even the most liberated woman wants to be treated with courtesy and respect.

It does not matter whether it's the woman or the man asking for the date; both are quite acceptable.

When the invitation is extended by the woman, she should be very clear that the date will be her treat. If she does not make it clear, the gentleman, when asked, should not be afraid to ask, "Are you asking me out as your guest?" If the answer is yes, or the answer is that she wants the two of you to go out and both pay, at least you know the terms of the request up front, from her response to your question, and you can proceed to respond with your decision.

Although the following features how to handle a date when going to a restaurant, the procedures are applicable for any and all other forms, such as: theatre; dance; drinks; bowling; or absolutely anything else.

Providing Date and Location

The host, whoever that is, should be completely up-front about all facets of the date. When and where are both very important when it comes to the other person accepting or rejecting the offer.

The time and location of the date is important because: they might already have something planned for that day and/or for that time; the location [or the event] may call for a level of attire [such as tuxedo for the man or floor-length gown for the woman] to which the person being invited may not be able to fulfill; if meeting at the venue, the guest might not have enough time between work and the designated time to go home and then to the venue. By providing the information up front, the decision, to accept or not, will be made based on all the parameters necessary to make an informed decision.

If the woman is the host, she should indicate what she feels appropriate when it comes to the start of the date. If she has a car and suggests she pick up the man, it is quite acceptable. On the other hand, if she does not have a car and asks if the man has access to one, and he does, it is her way of asking him to pick her up. He should proceed to pick her up.

Whether the man or the woman is driving, the gentleman should always handle the parking costs, unless the woman insists.

If the woman is the host and suggests that they meet at the restaurant, the gentleman should accept that without debate. The gentleman should arrive at the restaurant five minutes before the designated time. If his host is already seated, he should proceed to the table. On the other hand, if his host has not yet arrived, he should check his coat and wait for his host to arrive. When the woman arrives, offer to help her with her coat and then check it.

When it is time to proceed to the table, no matter who is the host, the woman should go first, then the gentleman.

Whether the woman or the man is the host, the rules of 'polite behaviour' still should be followed. The gentleman should open the doors; assist the woman with her coat and chair, etc.

The 'ticklish' part comes when it is time to order. Etiquette dictates that the host orders last and selects and orders the wine. A well-trained server should take notice as to who is ordering last and who is ordering the wine.

When the server presents the Wine List, it should go to the host. If the host is the woman, and the server starts to present the Wine List to the gentleman, the gentleman should merely state, "My host will be making that decision," and decline to accept the Wine List. If the woman specifically asks that the gentleman do the ordering, then he should accept the Wine List and proceed.

If the host is the woman, and the server asks her for her order ahead of the man, she should, merely, defer to the gentleman, which then sends a clear message to the server. Should the woman proceed to order first, the gentleman should, merely, acquiesce and accept the fact she has yet to read this 'Manual'.

When the server presents the bill, hopefully, they will have determined who is the host and place it closest to the host. It the host is the woman and the server goes to present it to the gentleman, the gentleman should, merely, smile and say, "This evening, I am the guest."

After you leave the restaurant, unless it has been discussed about going to another place, if the woman is driving, the gentleman should suggest that to save her having to go out of her way, he will take a taxi or public transit. By saying that, it offers the woman the choice of whether to accept his suggestion or to offer to drive him home.

If the woman drives the gentleman home, he has the choice of asking her in or saying nothing and merely treat the drive home as nothing more than what it was.

Follow-Up

After a date, if it was enjoyable, it is a much appreciated gesture to, either telephone the person the next day and tell them how much you enjoyed yourself, or email them within twelve hours and convey the same message.

If the woman was acting as the host, a nice gesture on the part of the gentleman would be to send her flowers to her work with a card enclosed thanking her for a wonderful evening. It need not be a lavish arrangement; it is the thought that is most important.

Handling A Bad Dating Result

Let's face facts; not every date is going to be fabulous. If you decide that you do not wish to pursue the relationship, be honest, but respectful.

Thank the other person for the opportunity to go out together; but, after giving it some serious thought, you feel that the chemistry is really not present. Wish them well and finish the call as soon after as possible. Never insult the other person or say hurtful things. It would be better to hang up [which is really something that should only be done as a last resort] than to get into a fight.

Handling Pressure To Be Intimate

If there is intimacy, it should occur naturally and when both participants are ready to proceed. Neither the woman nor the man should feel pressure to participate, or perform, until they are ready. If you are not at that point, say so. Do not be afraid to state your feelings and leave it at that.

If 'no' is disputed, merely use the door; and, realise that particular relationship was never meant to be.

TIPPING

The entire area of tipping is complex; and, must be viewed from the cultural, economical, practical and socially correct perspective.

Certainly, tipping in many cultures is considered de rigueur; yet, even then, will vary considerably. In Japan, for instance, tipping is considered offensive; whereas, in many others, you just might get spit at if you do not tip enough [think 'Paris taxi driver'].

Even when a 'Service Charge' is included in your bill, it is customary in some countries to add a few coins to 'top off' the tip.

In North America, a tip of 15% to 20% should be given. That holds true for foodservice, bar service, taxis, barbers, hairstylists, spa services, and all other services. Coat Check – $1 to $2; Door Attendants - $1 [if they hail a taxi add $1]; Bellmen - $2 per bag, minimum of $5; Room Service – if not already added to the bill – 15% - 20%.

Before travelling to a foreign country, always go online and check to find out what the correct tipping procedures are for the country. Make certain you have currency from that country with you, upon arrival, or visit an ATM as soon as you arrive at the destination airport. It is not courteous to tip people in a foreign [other than their own] currency; because, they will have difficulty exchanging it and, most likely, have to pay a premium do so. [Put yourself in their position – if you were providing that service in your country and they tipped you in a currency other than your home currency, you would be furious and offended.]

Also, whether you agree with the concept of tipping or you don't, stiffing [not tipping] a worker is not going to change the situation; it is just denying the worker the money they are counting on in order to take care of their family and themselves. One way or another, the worker, who is providing you a service, should be paid. Either it will be included in the cost of items, as in some countries, or it will not be and tips will be relied upon.

It always amazes me that many people will seek out the least expensive cruise or restaurant and then complain if a tip is included or they are expected to leave a tip. How do they think the cruise ship owners, or the restaurant owner, is able to offer such low prices. Of course they offer low basic wages and expect the tips to make up the difference. On expensive cruises, where tipping is not expected or required, the crew is paid much higher wages.

In other words, you cannot have it both ways. A worker is entitled to be compensated for services rendered. Therefore, if you don't like the concept of tipping, travel on more expensive cruise ships and only eat at restaurants where the prices include all service costs.

TRAVELLING – BEYOND YOUR COUNTRY'S BORDER

As an ambassador of your country, when travelling, your actions will, fairly or unfairly, directly reflect on your country and all of your fellow citizens.

For some, it is, sometimes, difficult to remember, because you are paying for the services, that you are still a guest in that country; and, you have been afforded the opportunity to visit the country as a courtesy.

If you still have difficulty understanding the dynamics, imagine you own a Bed & Breakfast that you and your family have spent a lot of money to promote. A family visiting from Russia arrive and ask if you have accommodation, to which you, gladly, answer, 'Yes'.

From that minute on, they snap their fingers at you and your family, demanding, usually in Russian, demands that you do not understand. Because you want them to like your country, you try very hard to make everything the best you can; but, no matter what you and your family do, it is not good enough; plus, they never offer even a 'Please' or 'Thank you'.

During dinner, they demand good, hearty, Russian food, instead of that terrible meal of locally raised meat and fresh vegetables your wife has prepared for them.

Before going to bed, they complain that the bed is improperly made and proceed to un-make the bed and demand feather duvets instead of the handmade patchwork quilt your great-grandmother made.

In the morning, they demand fish, cold cuts and cheese for breakfast rather than the home-made fresh croissants and jam, bacon and eggs and fresh fruit you and your wife had been preparing since 6AM.

The absolute capper comes when settling the bill they demand a discount from the price you had quoted and then pay you in Russian Rubles.

As unbearable as the above scenario would be, unfortunately, I have witnessed every single incident being perpetrated by tourists on the citizenry of various countries.

Rather than realise and accept that they have travelled to experience the differences, rather than the similarities, all too often, tourists behave like boors, talk down to the citizens of the country they are visiting, criticise everything, brag about everything back home and get totally offended when the people will not accept currency from, to them, a foreign country.

If you think it is always easy to convert money, just try, once you return home, to go to your local bank and attempt to exchange a small amount of any foreign currency, and if you can, not to lose quite a bit in the transaction. Good luck.

Next time, when you travel, before you become bellicose or short-tempered, try putting yourself in the other person's position. Enjoy the privilege being accorded you, respect their traditions and country, and use their currency.

I guarantee you will enjoy yourself more than you ever dreamt.

WEDDINGS - BRIDAL COUPLE

Bridal Registries

Using a Registry is a great convenience, especially for the guests. That may surprise you; but, today people are looking to make their lives easier and, also, save time.

When a couple registers at a store, especially one that provides a broad cross-section of important household items, such as china, flatware, decorative items, small kitchen appliances and kitchen incidentals, they allow the guests to easily fulfill their wedding gift buying.

Having been associated, for a number of years, with the world's greatest retailer of crystal, china, silver and gift ware, as well as their wonderful kitchen Gourmet Shoppe, I saw, first hand just how convenient a properly planned Bridal Registry can work, for both the Bridal Couple and the guests.

Being the originator of the Bridal Registry, almost seven decades ago, they constantly refined it to keep it current and convenient. The couples, who followed the professional advice provided to them, receive more gifts, especially gifts that they actually wanted, than couples who decided they knew better.

1. Register with only one store and make certain it can provide you with a full cross-section of primary household items. They should carry a broad assortment from major brands of: china patterns, silver and stainless flatware, crystal stemware, assorted decorative items and, if possible kitchen items [although the other items are the most important.

2. Many couples think they can register with a number of stores and 'force' their guests to buy them everything from luggage to bed linens and power tools. In reality, all they do is upset their guests and tick them off. Most guests want to be able to telephone, or go to, one store; be offered a number of choices within the price range they can afford and then buy. They will not run around in an attempt to satisfy your misguided demands. When you make it easy for your guests, they will buy you more and spend more.

3. Realise this is the one time in your life where you will receive the 'special items', such as good china, silver, crystal. If you don't go in this direction at the time of your wedding, because, at the moment, you are ambivalent about such items, ten to fifteen years from now, it will truly be regretted.

4. Register <u>before</u> you send out your invitations. Include an insert that shows where you are registered. [The store, with which I was affiliated, provided complementary inserts that were beautifully inscribed with the couples name, where they were registered, the store website address, telephone number <u>and</u> the address of the couple's <u>personal website</u>, which the store provided free of charge.

Invitations

Today, most people have very full schedules, with dates, months and years ahead. By sending out your invitations as early as possible, you guarantee that more of those invited will be able to attend.

Many years ago, inserting an insert explaining where you are registered was considered gauche. Today, it is considered a thoughtful act, which, merely, makes it easier for your guests to purchase a gift that will actually be useful and, therefore, kept.

If the wedding or the reception is being held in an unusual location, include an insert [so the guests can have it with them on the wedding day] that clearly provides directions [use Google Maps].

Include 'dress requirements'. That is achieved by indicating in the lower right corner [usually], Dress: Formal or Dress: Semi-Formal or Dress: Business or Dress: Casual.

In earlier times, an invitation would merely state, usually in the lower left corner, RSVP [and the address to which you wanted them to respond]. The response had to be an handwritten letter that followed a very specific content. I will not bore you with the contents; but, fortunately, today, life has become much easier. By including an insert that consists of a card, with the guest(s) name(s) and two boxes, ☐ Will attend ☐ Will be unable to attend, along with a Stamped, Self-addressed Envelope addressed, usually, to the Mother of the Bride.

Thank You Notes

Contrary to many ill-informed etiquette commentators, who mistakenly claim it is acceptable to send a 'Thank You' note up to a year after the wedding; a 'Thank You' note should be sent within one or two days of receiving either the gift or registry notice of purchase. By writing them on that basis, the task is not onerous and the 'Thank You' stays fresh and genuine, rather than banal and rote.

If gifts are received within a few days of the wedding, or at the wedding, the 'Thank You' should be written within two to three weeks of returning from the honeymoon.

Attire

As mentioned under Invitations, if you are planning for the wedding party to be attired in a specific fashion, you should communicate that to your guests, so they do not arrive being improperly attired. After all, as the hosts, you want your guests to feel truly welcome and comfortable. That will not happen if you are in Hawaiian beach attire and they are in tuxedo and floor-length dress.

Speeches

Make certain the person you have chosen to be the Emcee clearly understands your expectations. If he or she does not fully concur, thank them; but, select someone who does.

In today's 'anything goes' atmosphere, unfortunately some people feel it is appropriate to use the privilege of being asked to speak, as an opportunity to embarrass or, even, slander one or both of the bridal party.

Even if it is meant as humour, discussing previous relationships or even dates, is not appropriate. Neither is anything that may embarrass the bridal couple, the families of the bridal couple or, for that matter, anyone else. It is a day for compliments.

Humour, yes; hurtful comments or embarrassment, no.

Behaviour

It is unfortunate that I need to include this category; but, I do.

No one at a Wedding celebration, whether at the wedding location or the reception location, should behave, or be allowed to behave, in such a manner as to embarrass the Bridal Couple, their families, or, any other guests.

The Bridal couple should limit their alcohol consumption. Under the pressure of the moment, less alcohol than normally consumed may have a much stronger affect.

Excessive consumption of alcohol, by the guests, should not be allowed. The caterer should be told, when booking the facility, that you do not want anyone served more than they should have.

If anyone in the Bridal party, and I do mean anyone, has an habit of excessive drinking, they should be spoken to ahead of the day and asked to refrain from over-drinking. If you notice someone is beginning to have too much, have someone [not a member of the Bridal party] speak to them, somewhere away from the party.

Better to ask someone to leave than to have your special day ruined by an inconsiderate guest.

WEDDINGS - GUESTS

Invitation Acceptance

Upon receipt of a Wedding Invitation [or for that matter any invitation], speedy action should be given.

Delaying your response sends a message that you are holding off, in case a better offer might come along. You are either available for that date and you want to attend; you have something else scheduled for the time; or, you do not wish to attend. Determine which it is and return the 'RSVP' card as quickly as possible. Nothing is gained by delaying, except a bad reputation.

Gift

A client recently informed me that it was acceptable to send a wedding gift to the Bridal couple up to one year following the nuptials. Once and for all......that is not acceptable......by a long shot.

As soon as you respond, by returning the RSVP card, whether you are attending or not attending, you should proceed to purchase the gift.

If the couple is registered, purchase your gift from what they have selected.

[You would be amazed how often I have heard, 'I don't like anything they have selected,' or 'I don't like the china pattern (silver or crystal).' I hate to tell you; but, it doesn't matter whether you like what they have selected. It is not about you; it is what they selected; therefore, if you gift them with it, they will use it and enjoy it. Give them something not on their list

163

and they will, most likely, just return it if they know its' source or give it to someone as a gift.]

If the store has a 'Registry Notification System', let them take care of it; otherwise, deliver the gift.

In many cultures, traditionally, guests would bring their gifts to the actual wedding. In today's world, that is not practical. Weddings with hundreds of guests will mean there would be a mountain of gifts to handle. Items will be broken and stolen [believe me], or your card will get separated from the gift and the couple will never know who gave them the gift.

Save everyone, including yourself, a hassle; make sure the gift arrives as quickly as possible after you have responded.

When it comes to how much one should spend on the gift, the rule of thumb is you should spend, as a minimum, the amount the couple are spending to entertain you. Check to see where the reception is being held and then figure what you have heard is the going rate, including liquor. If a couple, double it.

Attire

Shocking as it is, some people who attend weddings feel a compulsion to out-dress the Bride, Attendants and the Mothers of the Bridal Couple.

The day is not about anybody other than the Bride and Groom; therefore, don't even think about turning your attendance into a competition.

Dress according to what the invitation indicates; or, dress according to the time of day. Use good judgement; but, remember to be understated.

Behaviour

Over-drinking; dancing on tables; scrapping with others; acting like a buffoon; doing a striptease; trying to seduce the Bride or Groom; etc., is not acceptable behaviour, no matter how much you think others will enjoy your actions.

Guests are in attendance to celebrate the Wedding Couple; and, as such, the party is, solely, about the Couple. Causing a distraction from them is rude and unforgivable.

FUNERALS

Overview

Many people claim they have difficulty 'handling a funeral'; and my question to them is, 'Is it really the actual funeral or is it your fear of dying?'

The good news is, if it is your funeral, you will not have anything to worry about; if it is someone else's, grow up and stop being self-centred. Attending a funeral is not in the least about you, other than affording you the opportunity to show how you felt about the person who has died; and, to show your support for the grieving family.

Concentrate on those objectives and you will be fine.

Flowers or Donation

Read the obituary, if possible, to find out what arrangements have been made and then respect them.

If you were merely a casual acquaintance, it is not expected or required that you send flowers, or make a donation to a designated cause. On the other hand, if you were close to the deceased, you may wish to carry out some gesture, to show your feelings, by sending a floral arrangement, either on your own or as part of a group. If you do decide to send flowers, the sooner the flowers are ordered the better. When ordering, have the florist read back to you what you have asked to be written on the enclosure card and ask the florist exactly when the flowers will be delivered. If there is a problem with either the card or the delivery time, speak up and let you wishes be known.

If you decide to make a donation to the designated charity, in the name of the deceased, do it when you are thinking about it; otherwise, you will, most likely forget about it.

Unless the obituary states that you may make a donation to the charity of your choice, respect the choice of charity, made by the family.

Visitation

Visitation, with either an open or closed casket, are not always assured; therefore, either check the obituary or call the Funeral Home and find out what hours, if any, are for the public. If you learn that the viewing is only for family, respect their wishes and do not attend. On the other hand, if there is a time allowed for the public; arrive no later than thirty minutes before the stated cut-off time.

Upon arrival, first sign the Guest Book, which is usually positioned just inside the entrance to the viewing room; and, then make your way to a family member, if you recognise any. If you do not, ask one of the Funeral Home attendants to point out one or more of the family.

Wait until the family member is available; then, if they do not know you, as you shake their hand, introduce yourself and explain how you knew the deceased. If you know the family member, depending on the local custom, kiss or shake hands.

Keep the conversation light and brief; if possible, relate some pleasant memory you have of the deceased. The family member may offer to take you to the coffin, if it is open; if they do, thank them and then accompany them. If they do not, take your leave and either make your own way to the coffin or quietly depart.

Throughout the time you are there, remember you are principally there to offer support to the family; therefore, refrain from getting maudlin; try to discuss happy memories; but, do so without becoming loud or obnoxious.

Funeral Service

You should be in your seat ten minutes prior to the posted start of the service.

Participate in the service to your level of comfort. If you are not comfortable with participating in a religious service, be courteous and stand and sit along with everyone else.

Internment or Inurnment

If the internment or inurnment is not posted as being 'Family Only', and you are a casual friend of the deceased, you do not have to feel that you need to attend. Usually, only close friends and family attend; but, it is quite acceptable for you to attend.

Upon arriving at the Funeral Home, prior to the service, let the attendants know whether you will be joining the funeral cortège. If you are, they will have you position your car, so that it will be easy for you to join the procession and, most likely, place a sign on the front of you car.

Once the cortège takes shape, maintain your position, as best as possible. Whether or not there is a police escort, unless the police are specifically stopping traffic at intersections to let the procession pass, you are legally obliged to respect all traffic lights and signs. If other drivers, as a courtesy, allow you to stay as a group, be very attentive at stop signs and traffic lights in case someone thinks they have the right-of-way.

Attending The Wake

If there is one, you are there to support the family and not eat or drink everything in sight. Enjoy but do not overstay your welcome.

INSIGHT

Obviously, there are thousands of situations involving etiquette and manners that have not been covered in this manual. Its' intent is to provide you with an overview of basic life situations and how you should apply manners and etiquette.

From there, extrapolate the lessons and apply them to events, as they occur, throughout your day-to-day living.

Above everything, live and enjoy an existence filled with courtesy towards all; it will return to you in un-told multiples, because people will respect you, want to be around you and want to see you succeed as you go from Clod To Suave.

Cheers,

Michael James Stewart
Image & Etiquette Coach/Consultant

<u>Now Available From Amazon.com & Other Retailers</u>

Faison Quay Mysteries

By

Michael James Stewart

Now That I'm Gone

~ First In The Series ~

Entrepreneurs, and wealthy in the extreme, Faison Quay VI and his partner, Dr. Stark Redfearne, take two of their closest friends and embark for South America aboard one of their company's cruise ships, only to have their plans quickly changed by a suspicious and disastrous event that resulted in death back in Toronto.

Upon proving it was a deliberate act, Faison engages his personal fortune and corporate resources to discover the "who and why" behind the crime. Each brilliantly uncovered clue allows Faison to peels-back another layer of craven hatred and deceit that led to the multiple murders, Now That I'm Gone.

In The Absence Of Passion

~ Second In The Series ~

Paris Police Inspector Gilbert Beaubien's frustrated efforts to solve the murder of an odious, yet famous, Louvre art restorer, is inextricably intertwined with world-renown, multi-billionaire, Toronto-based, Faison Quay VI, and his quest to locate the missing award-winning photojournalist, Passion Pomeroy, mother of Faison's son's fiancée.

Utilizing his vast wealth of contacts and money, Faison travels across Europe in his attempt to unravel the deepening mystery of Passion's disappearance and an increasing number of seemingly unrelated murders.

Fast paced and, oft-times, humourous, the story presents the reader with an abundance of clues, while informing and challenging them to solve the deepening mystery, In The Absence Of Passion.

Narcissus' Reflection

~ Third In The Series ~

Accused of systematically killing his family, Neith Donacon turns to the only person who believes in his innocence, David Granpré, Majordomo extraordinaire to world-renown, multi-billionaire, Toronto-based, Faison Quay VI.

David's unwavering belief is all that keeps Faison pursuing the truth when every new clue points assuredly at Neith.

Faison's quest takes him on a twisted, international, path of diamonds and demons; and, in the process, inadvertently endangers the lives of his family and friends.

The reader is once again treated to a multiplicity of clues that provide them with the opportunity to try to best Faison as he races to free Neith, by finding Narcissus' Reflection.

One By One

~ Fourth In The Series ~

A series of supposedly natural and accidental deaths causes the thirteenth Duke of Exeter to become a recluse and fear that he will be next to die. Each time he experiences chest pains, his doctor accuses him of imagining them or becoming a hypochondriac and his children are certain he is overreacting or, even worse, entering senility.

The arrival of his dear friends the world-famous Faison Quay, VI, and Dr. Stark Redfearne affords His Grace the opportunity to confide his fears to his guests and enlist their help in proving him correct.

Faison calls upon his wits and wealth to unravel the seemingly unrelated deaths and solve, before it is too late, why The Duke of Exeter's friends are dying One By One.

The First Stone

~ Fifth In The Series ~

Faison Quay's friend, Detective Sergeant Gregor Ferguson, of the Toronto Police Service, is assigned to investigate the body of a man, who had been missing twenty-seven years; but, just discovered in a garbage bin outside the Abbey of Perpetual Blessings. Suddenly ordered to stop investigating, Gregor asks Faison Quay if he will continue and involve the full force of one of his many companies, Key Security International, to assist. Faison Quay quickly discovers a web of nefarious situations that only he can bring to bay.

➡ ➡ ➡

Harcourt's Legacy

~ Sixth In The Series ~

Following the inaugural party of the supposedly impenetrable estate of Faison Quay scion, Faison Quay VII, fondly known as Veetwo, and his wife, Felicia, eight friends and family are abducted as they leave the estate. With no clues, and, seemingly, no reason behind the kidnappings, Faison mobilises his massive financial resources and staff.

When a number of employees of eponymous Key Construction are discovered murdered, Faison desperately attempts to determine if the deaths are connected to the abductions.

Eventually, Veetwo and Felicia, plus their entire staff, are forced to abandon their estate, which leads to the impossible occurring; in spite of totally being sealed to the outside world, the security of their home is compromised.
Faison races against all odds to unravel who is behind the crimes and what is motivating them, before the hostages are killed.

Perfection

~ Seventh In The Series ~

Several months after Pawel Piotrowicz, photographer extraordinaire and owner of the Picture Perfect Model Agency, was beaten and abandoned in a parking lot, by off-duty police, for having interrupted a Friday night drug-filled orgy, at Dr. Marshall Bendorff's Old Post Road mansion, and threatening to kill him for having performed cosmetic surgery on the perfect face of his client and world's top model, Vă; Piotrowicz was arrested and charged with the murder of Dr. Marshall Bendorff, owner of the world renown Yorkville area cosmetic surgery clinic known as Perfection.

When his lawyer, Barsla Panderric, is prevented from accessing the Coroner's and Police Reports, Pawel's discovery and friend, model and former Miss Black Canada, Ziam Ngout, implores her very close friend, Faison Quay VI, into proving Piotrowicz' innocence.

Utilising his resourceful and talented staff, at Key Security International, Faison unravels the seamy side of the doctor's life in an attempt to discover not only who killed him, but, how; as he uses his uncanny sleuthing abilities and phenomenal wealth to free Pawel Piotrowicz and prove Dr. Marshall Bendorff's murder was not Perfection.

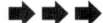

Final Curtain Call

~ Eighth In The Series ~

Two days after the opening, to rave reviews in a London revival, of Noel Coward's 'Private Lives', Dame Jocelyn Mahone disappears the same day her co-star and husband of thirty-one years, Sir Alistair Vickers, surprises her and the world, by announcing he is retiring.

Following a fortnight of inaction on the part of Scotland Yard, which feels it is a publicity stunt to boost ticket sales, Estelle Vickers, Dame Jocelyn and Sir Alistair's daughter calls the dear friend, Faison Quay, in Toronto, Canada, and asks for his assistance in locating her Mother.

Rather than merely having his famous Key Security International's London Agent take on the case, Faison, immediately flies to London on his private plane, along with his husband, Stark Redfearne, son, Faison Quay VII, affectionately known as Veetwo, Règinè Ouellette, Chief Operations Officer of Key Security International and former Commissioner of the Royal Canadian Mounted Police, and Faison's Personal Assistant, David Granpré.

Taking up residence in the Owner's Suite, of the six-star Key Hotel London, the world famous Faison Quay sets out to solve the mystery of Dame Jocelyn's disappearance, as well as two subsequent murders, before the Final Curtain Call.

Available In Soft Cover & eBook From
www.Amazon.com & Other Retailers

Website: www.MichaelJamesStewart.com

Email: Author@MichaelJamesStewart.com

Also From

Michael James Stewart

The Creator & Author Of
Faison Quay Murder Mysteries

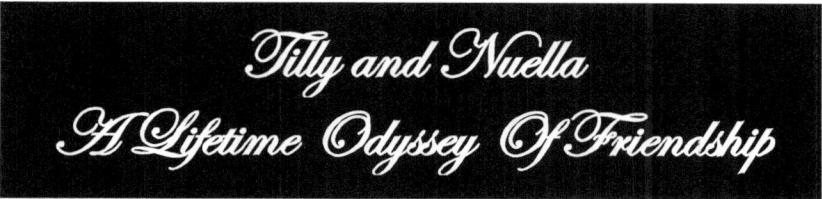

A beautiful narrative that bears witness to the fascinating lives of two young women, Tilly, from Lancashire in central England, and Nuella, from Northern Ireland, who, having fled their regional upbringing, strive to succeed beyond their humble origins.

Meeting just prior to World War II, in a London boarding house, both are resilient beyond their years and incredibly determined to create better lives for themselves and for those they come to love. Their innate decency continually plays them beneficial hands; from landing a job at the top secret wartime instillation of Bletchley Park to a post-war life, as war brides, in the burgeoning City of Toronto, Ontario, Canada.

Long after the novel ends, you will remember the epic friendship and journey of *Tilly and Nuella*.

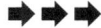

Available In Soft Cover & eBook From
www.Amazon.com & Other Retailers
Website: www.MichaelJamesStewart.com
Email: Author@MichaelJamesStewart.com

How Much Is Your Estate Worth?

For that matter, how much does anyone really know about you and your personal affairs? That doesn't mean you are expected to confide that kind of information to just anyone – but surely your husband, your wife, a child or your lawyer, solicitor, or attorney should be made aware of the whereabouts of your insurance, home and personal papers.

Okay, so they know you've made a will, signed a Power of Attorney – even prepaid your funeral. Good for you! Excellent!

BUT have you told anyone:

- Where you bank?
- Where your investments are?
- How about your insurance policies?
- And don't forget about your sources of income, as well as your debts and other liabilities pertaining to your estate.

Are Your Estate's Affairs Really in Order?

"Be Prepared" – the motto of the Boy Scouts, Girl Scouts and Girl Guides – has stood the test of time, been followed by millions of people, and should be a guiding light for everyone. Unfortunately, most of us continue to put off attending to anything that is even remotely associated with the possibility of becoming incapacitated (physically or mentally) and are no longer able or capable of taking care of our personal affairs and ourselves. Even more sobering – what will happen to those dependent upon us, or those we leave behind, when we die?

Obviously, no one likes to talk about death – even to think about it. Nevertheless, it doesn't do anyone any good to just bury their head in the sand, pretending it won't happen – because it will! And when it happens, will loved ones, significant others, relatives or friends know what to do?

Introducing an Estate Planning Tool

An excellent and helpful article in the Canadian senior citizens magazine, Good Times (Sept. 2001) dealt with this topic in a very general way when it advised its readers to "Share Financial Information; Introduce Professional Advisors; Assess Domestic Affairs; Prepare Contingency Plans and Take Advantage of Helping Hands." It is in that same spirit of helpfulness and "Be(ing) Prepared" that the comprehensive and detailed **Will and Estate Planning Inventory Kit** was prepared and is now available and useable to the general public, wherever they live throughout the world, with the hope that people will not procrastinate any longer, thereby taking the chance of leaving everything up to a spouse, lawyer, family member or friend to fret, worry and hunt for the many and sundry items, documents, information and property records that will be required by the various levels of government, care givers, etc.

Playing 'hide and seek' might be fun for kids – but it isn't fun for the person or persons left to finalize an estate and distribute various items – items that may or may not have been named in a formal will – items intended for 'specific' individuals. It is at that point where 'hide and seek' is no longer a game but instead, becomes a very real, serious and expensive business – expensive both in time and money. That's when the world's first, specially designed, comprehensive and inexpensive estate planning tool comes to the rescue!

Available In Soft Cover From <u>www.Amazon.com</u> & Other Retailers

www.ingramcontent.com/pod-product-compliance
Lightning Source LLC
Chambersburg PA
CBHW060304290526
45789CB00001B/398